The Biological Basis of Nursing: Mental Health

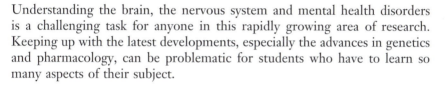

Understanding the brain, the nervous system and mental health disorders is a challenging task for anyone in this rapidly growing area of research. Keeping up with the latest developments, especially the advances in genetics and pharmacology, can be problematic for students who have to learn so many aspects of their subject.

Written by a nurse for nurses, *The Biological Basis of Nursing: Mental Health* brings biological and research information together. Generously illustrated, it provides a clear introduction to the workings of the brain, the nervous system and the underlying biology of mental disorders. It explains what happens in the brain in disorders such as schizophrenia and depression and lays the foundation for understanding why patients behave in certain ways.

This much, needed text prepares students and professionals alike for the revolution in pharmacology and genetics which is gaining pace every day.

Contents: introduction to the brain; neural communication; neurotransmitters and receptors; hormonal effects on mental health; genetic disorders affecting mental health; drug use and abuse; anxiety, fears and emotions; schizophrenia; depression; epilepsy; subcortical degenerative diseases of the brain; the ageing brain and dementia.

Dr William T. Blows, RMN, RGN, RNT, OstJ, BSc (Hons), PhD, is Lecturer in Applied Biological Sciences at St Bartholomew School of Nursing, City University, London. He is the author of *The Biological Basis of Nursing: Clinical Observations* (2001) also published by Routledge.

The Biological Basis of Nursing: Mental Health

William T. Blows

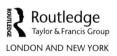
Routledge
Taylor & Francis Group
LONDON AND NEW YORK

First published 2003
by Routledge
11 New Fetter Lane, London EC4P 4EE

Simultaneously published in the USA and Canada
by Routledge
29 West 35th Street, New York, NY 10001

Routledge is an imprint of the Taylor & Francis Group

© 2003 William T. Blows

Typeset in 10/12pt Janson by Graphicraft Limited, Hong Kong
Printed and bound in Great Britain by TJ International, Padstow, Cornwall

British Library Cataloguing in Publication Data
A catalogue record for this book is available from the British Library

Library of Congress Cataloging in Publication Data
A catalogue record for this book has been requested

ISBN 0-415-24854-X (pbk)
ISBN 0-415-24853-1 (hbk)

Contents

Preface

The human brain is without doubt the most advanced organic structure ever to have evolved. Within this one organ reside our consciousness, cognition, thought, language, knowledge and learning, memory, emotions, perceptions, personality, behaviour, control of vital functions and movement, pleasure and pain. This is a staggering collection of functions, unequalled by any other organ. Without the brain we are nothing. It is the most precious item we possess.

Our mental health is dependent upon a healthy brain. In states of mental illness people are reduced to a minimal existence, robbed of their personality and shut away in a very different world from the one their body occupies. For many patients this is the result of disease, but for others it is the consequence of their own actions such as the deliberate administration of harmful drugs, or a head injury as a result of failure to wear a crash hat whilst cycling. Unlike general nursing where there is a need to reconstruct part of the body, for example a damaged limb, mental health nursing must attempt to reconstruct a damaged mind. This is made much more difficult by the complexity of mental illness and the fact that much is still unknown about it. Add to this the often-poor cooperation from the patient, and mental health nursing becomes a major challenge. The recovery process is long and tortuous, with progress limited in many cases. However, the more we understand of mental disorders the greater is the chance of success.

The mental health nurse requires a unique combination of disciplinary knowledge in order to provide a balanced and comprehensive scheme of care suited to each patient, including:

- an understanding of the concepts of psychology and psychiatry;
- a comprehension of the sociological aspects of mental ill health and its treatment;
- an ability to place the signs and symptoms of illness, and its therapies, within a biological framework of the nervous system.

This knowledge forms the basis of mental health nursing upon which the skills of the nurse are built. Whilst this book covers the biological components of mental health, it is essential for the student nurse to recognise the equal importance of the other scientific bases of care and to read this book in conjunction with those on psychology, sociology, the law and ethics and nursing practice.

The biology of mental health has had a difficult past, primarily because not very much was known about the brain in relation to mental ill health until thirty years ago. In addition, the introduction of the 'nursing model' in the 1970s and 1980s effectively did away with the notion that nurses should learn human biology. Anatomy and physiology were considered to be the doctor's domain and, in a desperate need for nurses to be seen as independent practitioners, anything resembling the doctor's training, especially biology, was either dropped from the curriculum or became a hidden curriculum. As a tutor in the 1980s, I remember a time when all anatomy sessions had to be labelled as 'nursing' on the timetable; for example, a session on the heart could not be entitled as such, but had to be called 'the nursing care of a cardiac patient', even though anatomy and physiology were taught during that session. Such were the extreme lengths we were forced to go to in order to sweep biology under the carpet. Biology was then, it seems, a necessary evil, and this approach has had unfortunate results. Whole generations of nurses qualified with less than adequate knowledge of how the body works. I recall one occasion when a consultant surgeon telephoned the school of nursing and complained that a senior student nurse did not know where the liver was. This situation was never destined to last, for two reasons. First, the practice of most nursing skills demanded some basic knowledge of the biology underpinning that skill; for example, some knowledge of microbiology is needed for the aseptic dressing technique, and some understanding of the systolic and diastolic readings is important for taking the blood pressure. This was essential if nurses were to understand what they were doing, why they were doing it and the possible outcomes of their actions. With the introduction of 'evidence-based practice', greater autonomy and accountability and the ever-extended role of the nurse, the understanding of biology has never been so important as it is now. Second, following on from the 'decade of the brain', research into both the functions of the brain and its disorders has reached global proportions. Huge volumes of new information are becoming available on neurology, genetics, neuropharmacology, biochemistry and other related sciences that will shape the pattern of treatment of both physical and mental disorders in the years ahead. If nurses are to remain participating practitioners in the delivery of care and treatment to the mentally ill, they must have at least some understanding of this research and its implications. Unfortunately, attitudes still exist where biology is placed outside the sphere of mental health nurses' needs. Ignoring or rejecting biology as a component in mental health nursing is at best backward looking and at worst damaging to the training needs of the modern nurse. Students trained with little understanding of the brain and its functions in mental disorder are ill-equipped to deal with what the future will bring in mental health.

This book identifies the major points the student needs or may wish to know from the massive amount of information on mental health biology now available. It provides a secure base for future exploration of the subject. It also serves as a reference book for qualified nurses in practice at all grades and for mental health nurse tutors who may not have fully developed the level of biological sciences needed to teach the subject with confidence.

There are some areas deliberately excluded from this book because they are considered irrelevant to the needs of the student nurse and would only serve to clutter the text with misleading information. The following areas are not included:

1 The techniques and methods of research, i.e. *how* the data was obtained. The methods used to investigate the brain can be found elsewhere if this information is required. Suffice to say here that most data is obtained by the standard means of post-mortem examination, various brain scanning techniques (MRI, PET, etc.), lumbar puncture, metabolic and blood flow studies, clinical trials, basic observations and physical examinations.

2 The thousands of scientific papers now available on most of the subjects covered in this book. Some key references that may be of particular interest are included. I considered that cluttering the text with hundreds of references would make the book tedious to read and would serve little purpose. The number of references on mental retardation is perhaps an exception and I have included a good number of these in a table for two reasons. First, mental retardation is a very important and interesting subject for the mental health nurse and I have tried to provide some opportunity for further reading on this subject. Second, I was surprised myself at the number of mental retardation syndromes associated with the X chromosome and I wanted to share with the reader some sense of the overwhelming volume of research and literature that exists in this area of mental health. Mental retardation offers one of the great challenges to mental health work at all levels, and that especially includes the parents of affected children.

As far as references are concerned, these are easily available on any medical and nursing subject through literature search lines or through the Internet. This is not specifically a pharmacology book, but I have tried to provide the basics that any mental health nurse should know about drugs, particularly drug abuse. However, the nurse should read this text in conjunction with a suitable neuropharmacology book.

The Biological Basis of Nursing: Clinical Observations (Blows 2001) was about the clinical skills of observations. The nature of mental health nursing is such that few clinical skills are actually discussed in this book. The administration of medication and the management of fits are the main skills highlighted. The real 'biological basis of nursing' here is the understanding of the science behind the illness, so that nurses have a better concept of the following topics:

• **The causes of mental health problems**, which is important in preventative care and in patient and family education
• **The pathology of mental health disorders**, which is important for understanding and participating in treatments, for giving information to

patients and relatives, and for the understanding of the outcomes of therapy, both beneficial and detrimental

- **The genetics, pharmacology and neurobiochemistry**, which between them are the future areas of development in mental health care.

These are the real skills of the mental health nurse in the years ahead, and the future mainstay of preventative and therapeutic care for the mentally ill.

Dr William T. Blows RMN RGN RNT BSc (Hons) PhD
City University, London
March 2002

Reference

Blows W. T. (2001) *The Biological Basis of Nursing: Clinical Observations*, Routledge, London.

Chapter 1

Introduction to the brain

Introduction

The human brain is one of Nature's greatest achievements. It is the development of the brain which has allowed humans to progress from their humble origins to putting a man on the moon. This chapter consists of an overview of the brain and contains many references to other pages where the area of the brain in question is explored further in more detail, usually in relation to a particular mental health pathology. At the simplest level the brain works something like a computer, but this is a computer like no other. It has been said that to build a computer to do everything the human brain does, the computer would have to be the size of Europe. Like a computer, the brain has an input (called a **sensory nervous system**) and an output (called a **motor nervous system**). Between these two systems, the brain carries out

cognitive functions, i.e. mental processing such as thought, memory and interpretation of the world about us.

As in a computer, things can go wrong; when they do, symptoms occur, just as with any other organ. The pathological conditions associated with the brain may be either **neurological** or **psychiatric**, depending on the degree of physical disturbance (neurological) or mental health disturbance (psychiatric) identified. These two types of brain dysfunction are becoming increasingly blurred as we learn that neurological conditions often involve disturbance of the mind and that mental health disturbance has some degree of physical (or biological) basis.

The brain can be divided into several developmental and functional areas as we move downwards from the top towards the base (Figure 1.1).

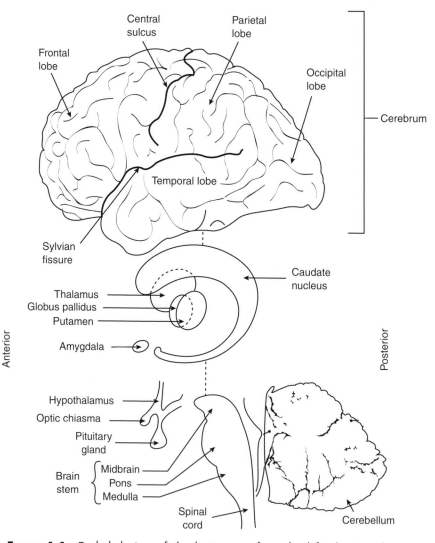

FIGURE 1.1 Exploded view of the brain seen from the left, showing the main components.

The **cerebrum**, at the top, is the largest and most advanced region of the brain, carrying out all our cognitive and conscious processes. Beneath this is the **limbic cortex** (cortex = surface layer), the area involved in preservation of both the individual and the species. This is the area involved in emotions, such as fear, and behavioural patterns, like eating, which are designed to keep us alive. Beneath this are the **basal ganglia** and the **cerebellum**, areas involved in control of movement at a subconscious (automatic) level. Finally, at the very base of the brain, the **brain stem** is involved in keeping the individual alive at the physiological level, controlling the heart, the blood pressure and the lungs amongst other functions (Martini 2001).

At tissue level, the areas of the brain are either **grey matter**, made from the cell bodies of **neurons** (brain cells), or **white matter**, made from the **axons** of neurons. Grey matter dominates the outer surfaces of the brain, with white matter inside. The surfaces are folded into **gyri** (singular **gyrus**, i.e. the top of a fold), and **sulci** (singular **sulcus**, i.e. the bottom of a fold) in order to increase the surface area for the purpose of packing in more neurons. Cell bodies which are separate from the main outer surface, i.e. patches of grey matter deeper inside the white matter, are called **ganglia** (e.g. the basal ganglia). **Nuclei** are patches of grey matter which have a specific controlling function (e.g. the cranial nerve nuclei of the brain stem). Several areas of the brain, such as the thalamus and hypothalamus, are actually discrete collections of distinct nuclei which are linked together by one name because they have similar, related functions.

See page 22

See page 11
See page 15

The meninges and cerebrospinal fluid

The brain and the cord are covered by membranes called the **meninges**, which form three layers (Figure 1.2). The innermost layer is the **pia mater** ('gentle mother'), the middle is the **arachnoid mater** ('spider mother') and the outermost is the **dura mater** ('tough mother'). Between the arachnoid mater and pia mater is the **subarachnoid space** containing a watery fluid called **cerebrospinal fluid** (**CSF**). This is formed from blood plasma inside the **ventricles** of the brain, i.e. the cavities within the brain substance (Martini 2001). CSF fills the two **lateral ventricles**, the **third ventricle** and the **fourth ventricle** before it flows out into the subarachnoid space. From here it circulates over the brain and cord surface before being absorbed back into blood via small projections of the arachnoid mater called **villi**. CSF also flows from the fourth ventricle through the **central canal** of the cord. CSF has several important functions.

1 It protects the central nervous system by acting as a water jacket, giving a cushioning effect to the central nervous system. This is a very important function, helping to reduce brain injury in accidents involving the head.
2 It provides support and flotation for the brain, which would otherwise weigh 30 times heavier without it!

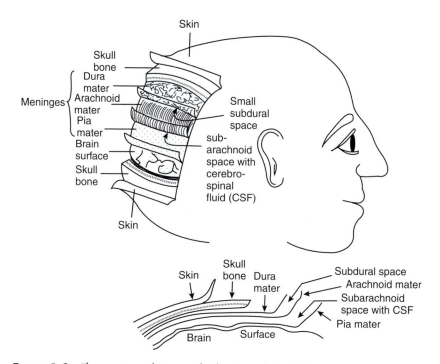

Figure 1.2 The meninges between the brain and the skull.

3 It delivers nutrition to some parts of the nervous system, since the CSF contains not just water but also some minerals and glucose.

4 It acts as part of an excretory pathway for the end products of neurotransmitter metabolism (known as **metabolites**) and some psychoactive drugs. These wastes pass from the brain into the CSF, then into the blood, which then goes on to the kidneys for filtering and the excretion of the wastes in urine.

CSF is often very important in mental health because of this role as an excretory pathway. One investigation, called **lumbar puncture**, is a method of collecting a sample of CSF in which the excretory products from brain chemicals or drugs can be measured. A needle is put into the spinal subarachnoid space below the level of lumbar vertebra 2 (L2) so as not to hit the solid spinal cord. The quantity of metabolite found in the CSF sample gives an indication of the amount of neurotransmitter that is active in the brain.

The cerebrum

The largest and uppermost area of the brain, the cerebrum (Figure 1.1), is divided into two **hemispheres**, left and right, each of which is further divided into four **lobes**. **Brodmann numbers** (Figure 1.3) form an internationally agreed numbering system to identify and map the major areas of the cerebral cortex according to their function.

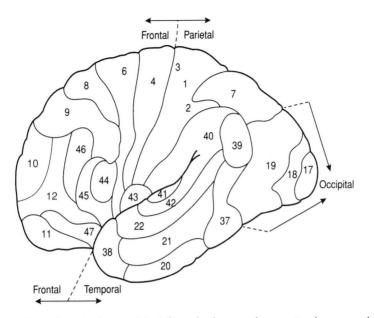

FIGURE 1.3 A functional map of the left cerebral cortex showing Brodmann numbers.

Frontal lobe

The **frontal lobes** contain the main **motor cortex** (motor = movement) (Brodmann 4) for each side of the body. Each cortex, left and right, controls skeletal muscles via long pathways descending into the spinal cord, then out to the muscles; these motor pathways are called the **pyramidal tracts** (Martini 2001). In addition, the **premotor cortex (**Brodmann 6), just anterior to the motor cortex, is involved in **motor planning**, a process that is vital for the swift and accurate execution of complex motor tasks. Speech motor areas (Brodmann 44 and 45), also known as **Brocha's area**, control the muscles of speech.

The frontal lobe also has areas concerned with the following range of important higher intellectual activities:

1 Achieving and sustaining attention and concentration;
2 Carrying out language activities, both spoken and in thought;
3 Maintaining memory;
4 Forming part of the pathways involved in emotions;
5 Carrying out complex skills involving visual space (i.e. **visuospatial tasks**) which require, for example, sequence planning or detailed copying of figures;
6 Performing **executive functions** such as monitoring one's own performance and making corrections as required, formulating and achieving goals, planning and reasoning.

The frontal lobes are the last part of the brain to mature, sometime after puberty, so teenagers function with reduced levels of emotional control and reasoning. The frontal lobes are the main centres of consciousness, particularly of self (i.e. self-awareness). Much of our **thought processes**, particularly **planning** (which requires forward thinking towards the future), reasoning and deduction, and many components of what we regard as our **personality** are due to the activities of the frontal lobes. It should therefore not be surprising to learn that many of the disorders of mental health either manifest within or involve the frontal lobes of the brain. Many of the symptoms we recognise as features of mental health disturbance, such as thought disorder or personality changes, may be traced to problems of the frontal lobes. No wonder that one of the very few psychosurgical operations carried out in the past for mental health reasons was a **prefrontal leucotomy**, which involved severing pathways leading from the frontal lobe to the other parts of the brain. Three main pathways involved in mental health disturbance connect the frontal lobe to deeper structures in the brain. These are the **dorsolateral** See page 19 **prefrontal circuit**, the **lateral orbitofrontal circuit** and the **anterior cingulate circuit** (McPherson and Cummings, 1999).

Parietal lobe

The **parietal lobe** involves the main **somatic** (i.e. from the body) sensory cortex (Brodmann 1, 2 and 3), and the somatic sensory association area (Brodmann 7). **Association areas** are essential for the interpretation, and therefore the understanding, of sensory stimuli. This is important because the brain is itself shut away from the world inside a bony box we call the skull. The only way the brain is going to know what is happening outside the skull is via the sensory nervous system, and by its ability to interpret those signals brought in by this sensory system. Association areas are therefore critical in the brain's understanding of the world around us. A language area (Brodmann 39, also known as **Wernicke's area**) is the main site for formulation of spoken sentences.

Temporal lobe

The **temporal lobe** houses the auditory area for the *conscious* sensation of hearing (Brodmann 41 and 42) and the auditory association area (Brodmann 22). What we actually hear is generated in the temporal lobe auditory area and not in the ears. Ears are organs necessary to convert sound waves into nerve impulses. The temporal lobe makes sense of these impulses as sound.

This lobe is also involved in the creation of personality and in emotional responses to sensory stimuli.

Occipital lobe

The **occipital lobe** has the main visual cortex (Brodmann 17) and the visual association areas (Brodmann 18 and 19) (Blows 2000a). This is therefore the *conscious* area for vision; that is, as with the temporal lobe and hearing, we actually 'see' the world with the back of the brain. The eyes only convert light energy into nerve impulses; it is the occipital lobe that makes sense of these impulses as a visual picture that we are aware of.

Functions

One of the most important functions of the cerebrum is the government of three important aspects of consciousness: awareness (sensory); cognition (e.g. thought); and response (motor). The entire cortex plays a role in consciousness, although for the most part the parietal, temporal and occipital lobes are involved with conscious interpretation of sensory stimuli, whilst the frontal lobe is concerned with consciousness of the 'self'. A discussion of consciousness and its relation to nursing observations can be found in *The Biological Basis of Nursing: Clinical Observations* (Blows 2001, chapter 7) (see also Blows 2000b).

The left hemisphere of the cerebrum is dominant for several functions, notably fine motor control, logic, analytical work, language and verbal tasks. Fine motor control means digital and hand movements, an essential part of many activities. Since most of the motor (i.e. pyramidal) fibres cross in the medulla, the dominance of motor control in the left hemisphere makes most people right handed. However, we know that it is entirely normal for left-handed people to be an exception to this, although left-handed dominance has not always been accepted by society. The right hemisphere is dominant for non-language skills, spatial perception and artistic and musical endeavours. People who have a general dominance of left hemisphere function are sometimes called *thinkers*, whilst those with right hemisphere function dominance are sometimes referred to as *creators*. This image of hemisphere functions may give the impression that the two hemispheres work in isolation. This is not true; they work together, communicating with each other through a bridge connection that joins the left hemisphere with the right hemisphere known as the **corpus callosum** (Martini 2001).

The basic functions of the brain in relation to some mental health disorders can also be reviewed in Silverthorn (2001, pp. 266–268).

The limbic system

The amygdala

The amygdala is a small pea-sized collection of nuclei situated at the tail end of the caudate nucleus (Figure 1.4). This tiny area is the emotional centre of the brain. It receives sensory input from several sources, particularly the cerebral cortex, the thalamus and the hippocampus (Figure 1.5) (Blows 2000c). Adverse stimuli from the external or internal environment of the body are known as **stressors** – potential threats to which the brain must respond with either an emotional or physical change. Output from the amygdala is to the brain stem (for emotional responses) and to the hypothalamus (for any physical response) (Figure 1.5). The amygdala is described in more detail in Chapter 7 in relation to emotions and phobic states.

See page 136

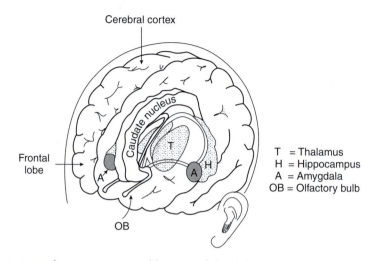

FIGURE 1.4 The components and location of the limbic system.

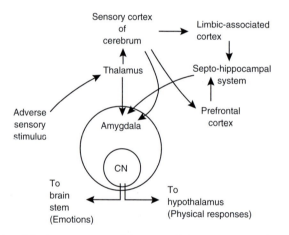

FIGURE 1.5 Simplified connections of the amygdala. CN = central nucleus.

The hippocampus

The hippocampus is tucked up underneath the temporal lobe of the cerebrum (Figure 1.6). The main function of this area is that of short-term memory, i.e. memory of very recent events (the last few hours), which will either be committed to long-term memory or forgotten (Blows 2000c). It is also involved in learning, which should not be surprising since learning is interlinked with memory. Emotional behaviour is also influenced by hippocampal activity, notably aggression. The hippocampus is described in more detail in relation to schizophrenia.

See page 148
See page 165

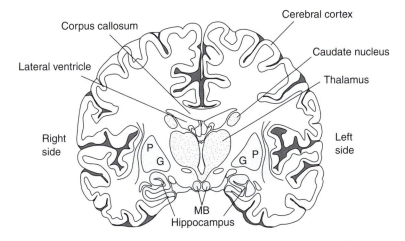

FIGURE 1.6 Coronal section through the brain showing the location of the cerebral cortex, the corpus callosum, the thalamus, the hippocampus, the mammillary bodies (MB) of the hypothalamus and parts of the basal ganglia. P, putamen; G, globus pallidus.

The thalamus, hypothalamus and pituitary gland

The thalamus

The thalamus is a collection of more than 30 nuclei situated underneath the cerebrum, close to the midline of the brain on each side (Figure 1.6) (Blows 2000c). The nuclei are set in four main groups: anterior, medial, midline and lateral. The thalamus is the *sensory relay station*; sensory impulses originating in the body (somatic) or the special senses (vision and hearing) pass into the thalamus, from where they are relayed to the appropriate part of the cerebrum. Visual nerve impulses from the retina must be relayed to the visual cortex of the occipital lobe (Brodmann 17, Figure 1.3), and nerve impulses generated from sound by the ear are relayed to the auditory cortex in the temporal lobe (Brodmann 41 and 42, Figure 1.3). Even somatic sensations from the body, e.g. touch or pain, are relayed to the appropriate part of the sensory cortex in the parietal lobe (Brodmann 1, 2 and 3, Figure 1.3). The sensory cortex has a cellular layout rather like a body plan, with cells in specific sites on the cortex accepting sensations from particular parts of the body. Impulses arising from the toes, for example, would be directed by the thalamus to the cortex occurring down the midline division, whilst impulses destined for the cells that accept sensations from the face would be directed to the lateral aspect of the cortex (Blows 2000b, p. 47). Pain is the only sensation that is 'conscious' at both thalamic and cerebral levels, whilst all other sensations must arrive at the cerebrum before we become aware of it.

The thalamus also focuses attention to specific sensations by making certain sensory areas of the cerebrum more receptive to sensory stimuli and other areas less receptive. Integration of some different sensory stimuli takes place inside the thalamus, a process essential for full appreciation of the information received by the sense organs.

The thalamus has a motor function as well. One particular thalamic nucleus links with the premotor cortex (Brodmann 6) of the frontal lobe, influencing motor function by increasing the focus of attention on the motor activity in progress. This influence is normally deactivated by the **basal ganglia motor loop** when no movement is happening, or activated when movement begins.

See pages 12, 13

The hypothalamus

The hypothalamus occurs as a collection of nuclei at the base of the brain (Figure 1.6) (Blows 2000c). These nuclei are arranged in anterior, posterior, ventromedial, dorsomedial and lateral groups. The **mammillary body**, a bulbous part of the hypothalamus, is a member of the posterior group of nuclei and a useful landmark on the undersurface of the brain. The hypothalamus is connected to the **pituitary gland** by a narrow stalk, the **pituitary stalk** (or **infundibulum**) (Martini 2001).

The hypothalamus has a wide range of functions and controlling centres:

See page 16

1 It is part of the **reticular formation** (see brain stem) that controls the **sleep–wake cycle**; the role of the hypothalamus is that of the **alerting centre**; that is, it wakes the brain from sleep by sending impulses out to the cerebrum.
2 It controls the body's temperature; that is, it is the **temperature regulation centre** keeping the body at 37°C. By monitoring blood temperature and acting as a thermostat it corrects the temperature if it goes too high or too low. The *anterior* part of the hypothalamus controls heat loss if the body gets too hot (e.g. by promoting sweating) and the *posterior* part controls heat conservation if the body gets too cold.
3 It regulates eating by giving a feeling of fullness (**satiation**), which prevents further food intake. This is the function of the **satiety centre** within the ventromedial part of the hypothalamus. Hunger and the seeking of both food and drink, however, are controlled by the lateral part of the hypothalamus.

See page 16

4 It controls the functions of both the **sympathetic** and **parasympathetic** components of the **autonomic nervous system** (**ANS**).
5 It influences sexual activity in combination with other regions of the brain.

See page 140

6 It plays a role in emotions.
7 It controls the hormonal output of the pituitary gland, both anterior and posterior lobes, by the following mechanisms.

Anterior pituitary lobe. **Releasing hormones (RH)** or **inhibiting hormones (IH)** (sometimes called releasing or inhibiting *factors*) pass down from the hypothalamus into the anterior lobe and either release, or inhibit the release of, the anterior lobe hormones. Anterior pituitary lobe hormones are:

- **growth hormone** – as the name suggests, it is important for growth;
- **adrenocorticotropic hormone** (**ACTH**), which acts on the adrenal cortex to stimulate the production of **cortisol**;

See page 140

- **thyroid-stimulating hormone** (**TSH**), which acts on the thyroid gland and causes release of the thyroid hormones T_3 and T_4; *See page 65*
- **prolactin**, which promotes breast milk production during breast-feeding;
- **follicle-stimulating hormone** (**FSH**), which stimulates the ovarian follicles to mature the ova (egg cells) in females and stimulates cells in the male testes to produce sperm;
- **luteinsing hormone** (**LH**), which promotes ovulation in females and stimulates the production of **testosterone** from the male testes.

Posterior pituitary lobe. The hormones that are released from the posterior lobe are produced in the hypothalamus. They pass down into the pituitary gland, where they are stored and released by hypothalamic control. These hypothalamic hormones are:

- **antidiuretic hormone** (**ADH**), from the **supraoptic nucleus** of the hypothalamus, a hormone which is released into the blood and acts on the **renal nephron** to conserve water;
- **oxytocin**, from the **paraventricular nucleus** of the hypothalamus, a hormone which is released into the blood and causes smooth-muscle contraction (for example, it contracts the uterus during labour), and also contraction of special breast cells which push milk towards the nipple during breast-feeding.

The basal ganglia and the cerebellum

These areas are part of what is called the **extrapyramidal tract** system; that is, they control the finer details of skeletal muscle movement at a subconscious level (Blows 2000c; 2001a, pp. 196–199). The extrapyramidal tract side-effects of drugs such as the antipsychotics are caused by disturbance to this system, particularly the basal ganglia.

The basal ganglia

The basal ganglia are made up of five main nuclei: the **putamen**, the **caudate nucleus**, the **globus pallidus**, the **substantia nigra** and the **subthalamus** (it is important not to muddle the thalamus with the hypothalamus and the subthalamus) (Figure 1.7). Several terms are used to describe the different ways in which some of these nuclei are grouped. The **corpus striatum** is the area involving the putamen and the caudate nucleus, with the main pyramidal motor pathways, called the **internal capsule**, passing between them. But the putamen is also part of the **lentiform nucleus**, which also includes the globus pallidus (Figure 1.7).

Collectively, the function of the basal ganglia is the fine control of muscle contraction (Martini 2001). The corpus striatum receives input from the main motor and sensory areas of the cerebrum, as well as inputs from the thalamus, subthalamus and the brain stem (particularly the substantia nigra).

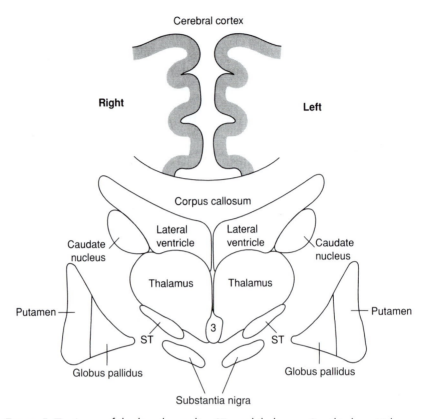

Figure 1.7 Areas of the basal ganglia. ST = subthalamus, 3 = third ventricle.

Output from the corpus striatum passes via the globus pallidus to the motor areas of the frontal lobe. The globus pallidus has several vital functions, notably the control of trunk and limb movements, including the positioning of limbs just prior to the movements of the digits, a function of the main motor cortex.

The globus pallidus and the putamen are also involved in the **basal ganglia motor loop** (Figure 1.8; see also Blows 2001a, pp. 198–200). When the body is not moving, the globus pallidus inhibits a particular thalamic nucleus which, when active, influences movement. As movement starts, stimulation of the putamen causes a blocking of the globus pallidus, removing the inhibition on the thalamus. The thalamus then becomes free to influence the main motor areas of the frontal lobe.

The substantia nigra is particularly important as the area decreasing **muscle tone**, the state of tension within a muscle, which is essential to achieve full contraction. The axonal tracts coming from the substantia See page 19 nigra to go to the putamen are the **nigrostriatal pathway**, and these use the See page 43 neurotransmitter dopamine. Degeneration of the substantia nigra causes See page 224 Parkinson's disease, and Parkinsonian-like symptoms are a feature of some See page 228 drug side-effects.

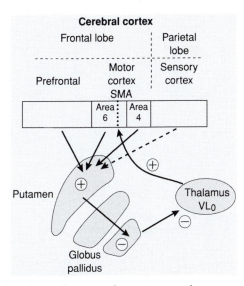

FIGURE 1.8 The basal ganglia motor loop. Input to the putamen comes from the frontal cortex, with less input coming from the parietal sensory cortex. This activates (+) neurons running from the putamen to the globus pallidus which, in turn, then deactivates (−) neurons linking the globus pallidus with the ventral lateral nucleus of the thalamus (VLo). These globus pallidus neurons were preventing (i.e. inhibiting, shown as −) any feedback from the VLo to the cerebral cortex. However, deactivation from the putamen has removed this inhibition, and the VLo then is free to feed back to the cortex (+) (more precisely, the supplementary motor area (SMA) of area 6 of the motor cortex).

The subthalamus has the role of inhibiting excessive motor activity from the cerebral motor cortex (i.e. acting as a breaking system for the pyramidal tracts). Disturbance of this function can result in excessive pyramidal activity affecting skeletal muscle contraction.

Apart from Parkinson's disease, disturbance of basal ganglia function includes several other different movement disorders, which are described in relation to psychotropic drug side-effects.

See page 175

The cerebellum

The cerebellum (Figure 1.9) is another part of the extrapyramidal tract system, controlling muscle function at a subconscious level (Blows 2000d). There are two hemispheres, rather as in the cerebrum, but just three main lobes: the **anterior**, **posterior** and **flocculonodular** lobes. Each lobe is further subdivided into smaller regions of surface area. This surface is made of grey matter, which is folded to increase the area to about 75% of the surface area of the cerebrum. There is white matter below the surface and at the core of this white matter are further patches of grey matter, the **cerebellar nuclei**. The routes for impulses to pass into and out from the cerebellum are through the brain stem via the **cerebellar peduncles**, foot-like connections between the cerebellum and the brain stem (Martini 2001).

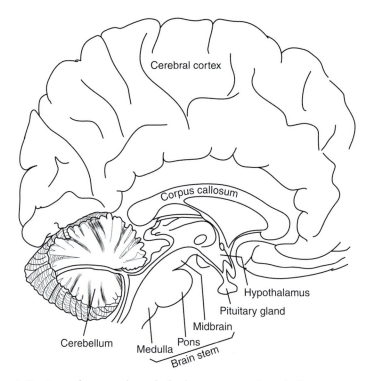

FIGURE 1.9 Sagittal section through the brain stem and cerebellum.

The functions of the cerebellum are as follows:

1 To maintain the balance of the body. The cerebellum makes fine adjustments to muscle tensions to stabilise body position, especially when upright, to prevent falling over. Sensory feedback on balance, to the cerebellum, is from somatic **proprioception** (sensory information on body position from muscles, tendons and joints), and **vestibular** information from the semicircular canals of the inner ear. The proprioception impulses enter the anterior lobe of the cerebellum, whilst vestibular impulses pass into the flocculonodular lobe.

2 To smooth out muscle movement, preventing erratic movements and facilitating fine, well-controlled movements.

See page 12

3 To increase muscle tone in opposition to the substantia nigra.

4 To effect *synergy*, i.e. a collection of different muscle movements made simultaneously to achieve a particular objective. The cerebellum creates a motor plan, whereby multiple muscles function together in one activity. A good example is the coordination required to catch a ball which is moving towards you. Visual information on the nature of the object, its speed and direction, is flashed to the cerebellum. The entire muscle sequence needed to catch the ball is planned, slightly ahead of time (to allow for movement of the ball whilst planning and muscle movement takes place), and the activity is then executed.

These skills are not present in the newborn infant. The cerebellum has to learn, by trial and error, to balance the body, smooth and coordinate muscle activity and to interact with moving objects. Parents can often identify the moments in the development of a child when the cerebellum achieves a new skill, such as the first moment the infant stands unsupported, balancing on both legs. Repeated attempts at a skill improve the cerebellum's ability to learn and perfect that skill. *Practice makes perfect* could be rewritten to read *practice makes better cerebellar function*.

The brain stem

This part of the brain is the most primitive in that it carries out the basic functions of living (Blows 2000d). It is the lowest area of the brain (Figure 1.9) and is continuous with the spinal cord. The distinction between brain stem above and cord below is approximately at the level of the **foramen magnum**, the 'large window' at the base of the skull.

The brain stem is divided into three parts, the uppermost part being the **midbrain**. Below this and bulging anteriorly is the **pons**, and the lowest part is the **medulla** (Figure 1.9). The pons is often referred to as *bulbar*, meaning it is swollen like a bulb. The brain stem houses many nuclei, a large number of which are those that control the functions of most of the 12 pairs of **cranial nerves** (numbers **III** to **XII**). Cranial nerves are the nerves that come direct from the brain. Cranial nerves I (olfactory) and II (optic) come from the brain at a higher level than the brain stem.

The midbrain is the smallest part of the brain stem, just above the pons. Here cranial nerve nuclei numbers III (oculomotor) and IV (trochlear) are found. These nerves and their nuclei are concerned with eye movements.

The pons has cranial nerve nuclei numbers V (trigeminal), VI (abducent), VII (facial) and VIII (vestibulocochlear). Two other nerve nuclei are part of the respiratory control centres shared with the medulla.

The medulla is the lowest part of the brain stem. The remaining cranial nerve nuclei are found here with their associated nerves: IX (glossopharyngeal), X (Vagus), XI (accessory) and XII (hypoglossal). The medulla also contains the vital centres which keep the body alive: the **cardiac centre** essential for heart function, the **respiratory centres** (shared with the pons) which together keep the individual breathing, and the **vasomotor centre** (**VMC**), a diffuse set of nuclei which collectively influence peripheral vascular resistance, part of the mechanism for maintaining blood pressure. The medulla is also the location for a number of reflexes which, again, are primitive responses to stimuli designed to protect the body against harm or even death. Such reflexes include the **gag reflex** (which prevents unwanted substances from entering the throat), the **corneal reflex** (which prevents injury to the front of the eye by shutting the lids if something touches the eye), and the **pupillary reflex** (which shuts down the pupil in bright light, preventing light-induced retinal injury). Some of these reflexes are used in neurological investigations to assess brain stem function.

Parts of the medulla, the pons, the midbrain and the upper cord contain discrete patches of small nuclei, which collectively are referred to as the

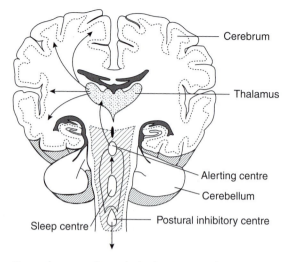

Figure 1.10 Coronal section through the brain stem showing area of the reticular formation (shaded) and the main centres of the sleep–wake cycle. Impulses from these centres are distributed either to the cortex via the thalamus or to the body via the spinal cord, as shown by the arrows.

reticular formation (**RF**) (Figure 1.10) (Blows 2000d). These nuclei have connections with many parts of the brain. The reticular formation has the role of inhibiting those sensory stimuli entering the brain that can be considered as repetitive, weak or unnecessary, allowing only strong, significant or unusual impulses to pass. Other mechanisms such as vomiting, swallowing, coughing and sneezing are brain-stem RF-mediated functions, and are all linked to the function of respiration in some way. Part of the RF is the **reticular activating system** (**RAS**), i.e. those RF components that are responsible for the **sleep–wake cycle**. This cycle controls the timing of sleep in relation to light levels falling on the retina. The RAS has an **alerting centre**, part of the hypothalamus that sends out impulses to the conscious brain in order to maintain alertness when awake. The RAS also has a **sleep centre** lower down in the brain stem, which causes sleep through impulses sent to the conscious brain (cerebrum) via the thalamus. There is also a **postural inhibition zone** at the lowest point of the brain stem where it meets the cord (Figure 1.10). This zone blocks muscle activity during sleep by sending inhibitory impulses down through the cord to the muscles in order to prevent individuals from acting out their dreams. Disturbance of the RAS is likely to cause abnormal changes in the sleep pattern associated with several mental health disorders.

See page 32

The autonomic nervous system

The autonomic nervous system (ANS) is that part of the peripheral nervous system that functions automatically, i.e. without conscious control. The two parts of the ANS are the **sympathetic** and **parasympathetic** systems

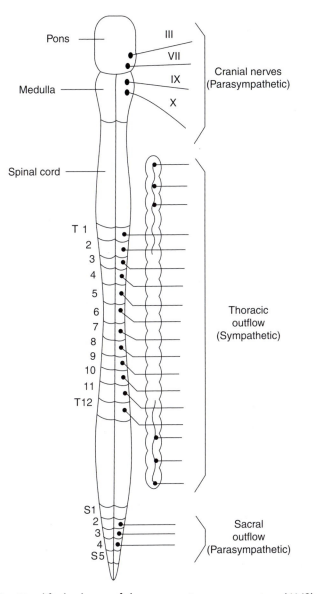

FIGURE 1.11 Simplified scheme of the autonomic nervous system (ANS). Cranial nerves (III, VII, IX and X) are shown in roman numerals. T = thoracic, S = sacral.

(Figure 1.11; see also Blows 2001b, p. 43). They act between them to stabilise many physiological parameters (for example, heart rate is stabilised at an average of 72 beats per minute), but the two parts allow the parameters to change when it becomes appropriate (for example, the heart rate can increase or decrease depending on the circumstances). The sympathetic component serves to increase those parameters useful for reactions to adverse stimuli, such as fear. Responses to stimuli like fear result in, amongst other things, fast pulse rates, sweating and increased respiration, all of which are

See page 146

TABLE 1.1 Functions of the autonomic nervous system

Target organ (or system)	Sympathetic function	Parasympathetic function
Mental alertness	Increases	No effect
Eye (pupil)	Dilates	Constricts
Heart muscle	Increased heart rate and force of contraction	Decreased heart rate
Coronary arteries	Dilated	Constricted
Blood pressure	Raised	Lowered
Bronchi	Dilated	Constricted
Digestive tract	Reduced peristalsis and increased sphincter tone	Increased peristalsis and decreased sphincter tone
Stomach	Reduces digestion	Increases hydrochloric acid
Liver/blood glucose	Glucose released from glycogen into blood	No effect
Kidney	Decreased urine produced	No effect
Bladder	Allowed to fill, internal sphincter closed	Emptied, sphincter opened
Adrenal medulla	Releases adrenaline	No effect
Metabolism	Increased	No effect
Skin	Increased sweating	No effect

important in speeding up oxygen delivery to the tissues for a response to the cause of the fear. The parasympathetic component causes an opposite effect by reducing the physical parameters, e.g. slower heart and breathing rates, at times of rest. The range of functions for each system can be seen in Table 1.1.

Table 1.1 illustrates the balance effect of the two systems working together to give *average* parameters, but averages that can shift in either direction as circumstances dictate. For example, heart rate averages at about 72 beats per minute but can rise to 120 or more in exercise or anxiety, or fall towards 60 during complete rest. Excessive sympathetic activity is seen in anxiety and phobic states when patients come into contact with their fears. Some parameters do not have an opposing parasympathetic activity.

See page 146

The main pathways involved in mental health

Table 1.2 (Figure 1.12) shows the pathways of the brain that are chiefly involved in mental health disorders, **psychotrophic** (affecting the mind) drug activity and drug side-effects. Further discussion of the pathways (or tracts) is given under the relevant neurotransmitter (Chapter 3), under the appropriate disorder and under the pharmacology involved.

TABLE 1.2 Brain pathways involved in mental health

Pathway	Figure numbers	From	Pathway To	Importance to mental health	
Mesolimbic pathway	1.12, 3.5, 8.5	Brain stem	Limbic system	Probably involved in psychotic symptoms, e.g. schizophrenia	*See pages 175, 177*
Mesocortical pathway	1.12, 3.5, 8.5	Brain stem	Cerebral cortex	Probably involved in psychotic symptoms, e.g. schizophrenia	*See page 177*
Nigrostriatal pathway	3.5, 11.2	Substantia nigra	Corpus striatum	Site of extrapyramidal side-effects of drugs and of Parkinson's disease	*See page 176*
Diffuse modulatory systems	3.6, 3.7, 9.3	Brain stem	Many parts of limbic area and cerebral cortex	Appears to be involved in depression and possibly eating disorders	*See page 184*
Median forebrain bundle	4.1	Brain stem	Frontal lobe of cerebrum	Involved in the brain reward pathways which are implicated in drug addiction	*See page 114*
Dorsolateral prefrontal circuit		Frontal lobe (Brodmann 9 and 10)	Head of caudate nucleus (basal ganglia)	Involved in deficits of frontal lobe executive functions	
Lateral orbitofrontal circuit		Prefrontal cortex (Brodmann 10)	Caudate nucleus	Involved in mood and personality changes	
Anterior cingulate circuit		Anterior cingulate gyrus (Brodmann 24) of the frontal lobe	Several areas of brain stem and basal ganglia	Involved in speech and emotional loss, and apathy	

Key points

The meninges and cerebrospinal fluid

- The brain and the cord are covered by the meninges in three layers: the pia mater, the arachnoid mater and the dura mater.
- Between the arachnoid mater and pia mater is the subarachnoid space containing cerebrospinal fluid (CSF).
- Two lateral ventricles, the third ventricle and the fourth ventricle inside the brain are filled with CSF.
- CSF has several functions, such as protection of the central nervous system, support and flotation for the brain and possibly nutrition, and is part of the excretory pathway for the brain. For example, it is a major

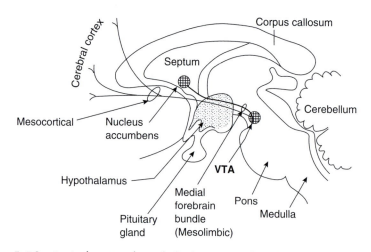

FIGURE 1.12 Sagittal section through the brain stem showing the ventral tegmental area (VTA) and the main dopaminergic pathways; the mesolimbic pathway (through the medial forebrain bundle) and the mesocortical pathway.

excretory pathway for many psychoactive drugs and neurotransmitter metabolites.

- Lumbar puncture is a method of collecting a sample of CSF from the subarachnoid space below the lumbar vertebra 2 (L2) level.

The cerebrum

- The cerebrum is the largest part of the brain, carrying out our cognitive and conscious processes.
- The frontal lobe is a major part of the brain involved in many mental health functions; in particular it is the site of consciousness of the 'self'.

The limbic system

- The limbic system below the cerebrum is involved in preservation of the individual and the species, and involves emotions and controlling behavioural patterns.
- The amygdala is the emotional centre of the brain.
- The function of the hippocampus is in short-term memory, learning and emotional behaviour.

The thalamus and hypothalamus

- The thalamus is the sensory relay station, passing sensations to the cerebrum.
- The hypothalamus has a wide range of functions, notably temperature control, regulation of eating, alerting the brain after sleep and

controlling the pituitary gland's hormones and the autonomic nervous system.

The basal ganglia and the cerebellum

- Below the limbic area are the basal ganglia and the cerebellum, areas involved in control of movement at a subconscious level (i.e. part of the extrapyramidal tract system).
- The function of the substantia nigra is the reduction of muscle tone.
- The functions of the cerebellum are fine control of balance, smoothing out muscle movement and synergy.

The brain stem

- The brain stem has the nuclei that control the cranial nerve functions and the vital centres, such as respiration, cardiac function and blood pressure. It also has the reticular formation and the reticular activating system that controls the sleep–wake cycle.

References

Blows W. T. (2000a) The nervous system, part 1. *Nursing Times*, **96** (35): 41–44.

Blows W. T. (2000b) The nervous system, part 2. *Nursing Times*, **96** (40): 45–48.

Blows W. T. (2000c) The nervous system, part 3. *Nursing Times*, **96** (44): 45–48.

Blows W. T. (2000d) The nervous system, part 4. *Nursing Times*, **96** (48): 47–50.

Blows W. T. (2001a) *The Biological Basis of Nursing: Clinical Observations*. Routledge, London.

Blows W. T. (2001b) The nervous system, part 7. *Nursing Times*, **97** (10): 41–44.

Martini F. H. (2001) *Fundamentals of Anatomy and Physiology* (5th edn). Prentice Hall, Upper Saddle River, NJ.

McPherson S. E. and Cummings J. L. (1999) The neuropsychology of the frontal lobes *in* Ron M. A. and David A. S. (eds), *Disorders of Brain and Mind*. Cambridge University Press, Cambridge.

Silverthorn D. U. (2001) *Human Physiology, An Integrated Approach* (2nd edn) Prentice Hall, Upper Saddle River, NJ.

Chapter 2

Neural communication

- The neuron
- Neurotransmission
- Synapses
- Neuroglia
- Key points

The neuron

The functional unit of the nervous system is the neuron (Figure 2.1). All nerve impulses, or **action potentials**, originate in neurons. They travel along the neuron's extended cytoplasm, called the **axon**, to the point inside or outside the brain where an impulse is required to initiate one of many possible actions – for example, triggering another action potential within a second neuron, or a muscle contraction, or possibly a glandular secretion. Action potentials make things happen and therefore the cell generating the impulse has some control over that action. Strong or rapidly repeated impulses along a neuron result in powerful activities, such as muscle contraction.

We are born with 100 billion neurons, an amazing number by any standards, yet this vast mass of cells constitutes only about 10% of the entire nervous system. The remaining 90% is made up of 900 billion glial cells (also known as **neuroglia**), which have very different functions from neurons. There is a grand total of 1000 billion cells in the nervous system, all derived from the same single fertilised ovum as the rest of the body. A very high rate of cell mitosis is required *before birth* to produce this vast number of neurons, about 250 000 new neurons *per minute*! Although recent

See page 34

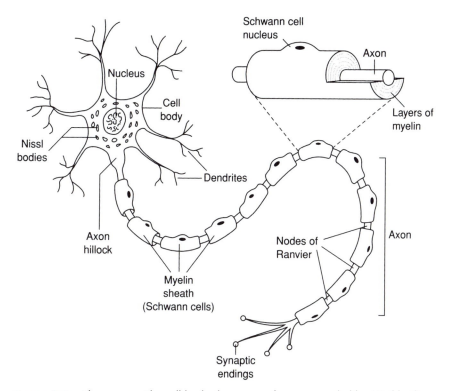

FIGURE 2.1 The neuron. The cell body shows a nucleus surrounded by Nissl bodies. The axon starts at the axon hillock and terminates at the synapse. Myelin covers the axon in segments with gaps between called the nodes of Ranvier. A myelin segment is shown enlarged. Each segment is laid down by a Schwann cell.

evidence indicates that some neuronal division can occur after birth (Day 1997), the neuron cell mass is essentially complete at the time of birth. However, the neuronal connections, called **synapses**, are not complete. They continue forming throughout childhood until the brain becomes fully mature in the late teens or early twenties. Synaptic development in childhood is promoted by stimulation of the senses and by education, and involves the creation of memory.

See page 244

In general, maturation of the brain is based on three stages of neuronal development:

1 neuronal migration;
2 neuronal myelination;
3 neuronal connections (synapses).

See page 168
See page 36
See page 30

However, many *neuroglia* retain the power to replicate after birth and continue to do so throughout life.

The neuron (Figure 2.1) has a relatively standard cell body, with a surrounding cell membrane, a cytoplasm with **organelles** such as **mitochondria** (for cellular energy) and **ribosomes** (for producing proteins), and a nucleus with its own nuclear membrane. It is distinguished from other cells by the presence of cell body extensions, called dendrites and axons, and **Nissl granules** (or **Nissl bodies**) within the cytoplasm.

Dendrites are mostly *afferent* pathways; that is, they convey impulses *towards* the cell body. There are usually many such dendrites, branching in a number of different directions, each branch covered by short processes called spines. The more dendrites or dendritic spines a neuron has, the greater is the surface area available for forming synaptic connections. Dendrites are the sites of many synapses, which are formed from the local connections they have with other neighbouring neurons. **Axons** are *efferent* pathways, carrying impulses *away from* the cell body. Most neurons have only one axon, but there are examples of neurons with more than one. They can be long – some are nearly the length of the body – and they have few branches except at the terminal end. The majority of neurons are myelinated and they make distant connections with other neurons, muscle cells or glandular cells (Blows 2000).

Nissl granules (or Nissl bodies) are patches of intracellular **rough endoplasmic reticulum** (**rough ER**) and are the site of protein synthesis carried out by **ribosomes** (protein factories) in the ER membrane. Nissl bodies are especially concentrated close to the nucleus, in the region of the cytoplasm known as the **endoplasm**. Proteins produced in Nissl bodies are used within the cell to create membranes or organelles.

Axoplasmic transportation

Proteins are also required at the synapse, the terminal end of the axon, but because ribosomes are not found in the axon they must be transported there from their source within the cell body. This **axoplasmic transport** (Figure 2.2) of proteins is a function of part of the cell's **cytoskeleton**; the protein

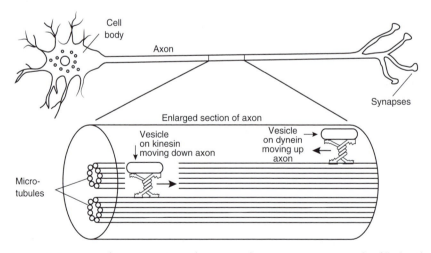

FIGURE 2.2 Axonal transportation. The protein kinesin transports vesicles filled with other proteins along microtubules towards the synapse. Another protein called dynein does the same in the opposite direction.

support framework of the cell. Three structures are involved in this framework: **microtubules** (20 nm in diameter), hollow tubules made from the protein **tubulin** (see also Alzheimer's disease); **microfilaments** (5 nm in diameter), cable-like structures made from two twisted proteins; and **neurofilaments** (10 nm in diameter), strong structures branching out in many directions. Like the bony skeleton inside the body, this protein framework of the cell provides shape, support and some movement to the neuron, as well as allowing the mechanism of axoplasmic transport.

See page 251

Axoplasmic transport first involves the packaging of essential proteins into vesicles that are destined for the synapse. These vesicles are then attached to another protein called **kinesin**. Using cellular energy in the form of **adenosine triphosphate** (**ATP**), produced by another organelle, the **mitochondrion** (Blows 2001, chapter 1), the kinesin moves down the axon. Kinesin acts like legs to 'walk' the vesicle along the microtubules, which extend in bundles along the full length of the axon. In the long journey to the synapse, two speeds of axonal transportation have been observed. **Slow transportation** moves the vesicles up to 10 mm per day, while **fast transportation** moves them up to 1000 mm (1 meter) per day. This is **anterograde** movement, i.e. from cell to synapse, involving the transportation of some neurotransmitters, but **retrograde** movement also occurs, from synapse to cell body, using the protein **dynein** in place of kinesin. Retrograde axoplasmic transport may be involved in feedback to the cell body related to the protein needs of the synapse (Figure 2.2). The whole axoplasmic transportation system is akin to the movement of goods by train along fixed tracks. It is important not to confuse axoplasmic transportation (protein movement along axons) with **neurotransmission** (the passage of an electrical impulse along axons). Understanding neurotransmission is vital in grasping the main concepts of how the brain works and how drugs can modify its function.

Neurotransmission

Resting potential

Neurotransmission is the passage of a nerve impulse (or **action potential**) along a neuronal axon. Before and after an action potential, the membrane is said to be in **resting potential** (Figure 2.3). Resting potential involves a very distinct concentration of **ions** on both sides of the membrane. Ions are charged particles, either positively charged (+) particles called **cations**, or negatively charged (−) particles called **anions**. The particles themselves are atoms of elements like sodium (forming a cation, Na^+), potassium (forming a cation, K^+), or chloride (forming a chloride anion, Cl^-). The ionic concentrations on both sides of the axonal membrane are shown in Figure 2.3. There is a sodium concentration outside the membrane (i.e. in the extracellular fluid), and a potassium concentration inside the membrane (i.e. in the cell cytoplasm). In addition to ions, there are compounds that also carry an electrical charge, notably proteins and phosphates (PO_4), both of which have three negative charges each. Because of their large size, these compounds

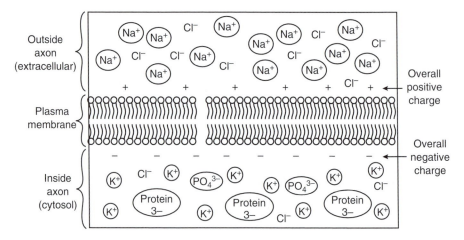

FIGURE 2.3 Resting potential in the neuronal membrane. Outside the membrane is a concentration of sodium, whilst inside is a concentration of potassium. The overall charge outside is caused mostly by the sodium, whilst the inside is negative because large negatively charged protein and phosphate (PO_4^{3-}) molecules cannot leave the axon.

cannot pass through the membrane and are therefore confined to the cytoplasm inside the membrane. If all the charges on each side of the membrane are added together (with each negative cancelling a positive), the net charge which remains after such cancellation is negative on the inside and positive on the outside. The *difference* between this overall negative charge *inside* the membrane and the overall positive charge *outside* the membrane is minus seventy thousandths of a volt (**–70 mV**, or minus seventy millivolts). This is the electrical value for the resting membrane potential.

Diffusion

The membrane of the neuronal axon is semipermeable and as such it allows the occasional passage of ions one way or another. Sodium, for example, may tend to leak inwards, moving down its concentration gradient from a high concentration outside to a low concentration inside. Potassium on the other hand, moving down its concentration gradient, may leak a little in the opposite direction. This is a natural movement for particles, which pass from a high to a low concentration in an attempt to equalise the concentration on both sides of the membrane (the process of **diffusion**). Diffusion of particles is the driving force for the movement of many substances both into and out of cells in many parts of the body.

Threshold potential

While leakage causes small fluctuations to occur in the resting potential of –70 mV, an action potential delivered from elsewhere will cause a rapid change. In fact, as soon as the resting potential reaches –50 mV, a rapid

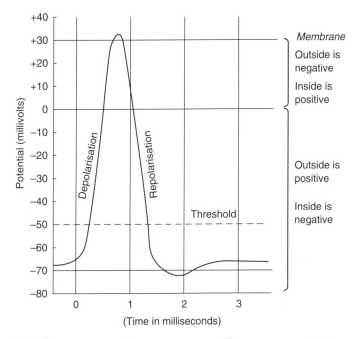

FIGURE 2.4 The action potential as seen on an oscilloscope screen. Resting potential is –70 mV. If sufficient depolarisation occurs for this value to reach –50 mV (threshold), an action potential will take place. Depolarisation is caused by sodium influx until +30 mV is reached. Repolarisation then occurs with a potassium efflux until resting potential is restored. As depolarisation and repolarisation cross 0 mV so the net charge on each side of the membrane reverses.

opening of sodium channels in the membrane allows a massive influx of sodium into the axon, creating a new action potential. This figure of **–50 mV** is called the **threshold potential** (Figure 2.4), and marks the opening of many sodium channels in the membrane. The sodium floods into the axon because, as a positive ion, it is attracted to the overall negative charge on the inside of the membrane (an electrical effect). Also, it will move rapidly down its concentration gradient (a chemical effect). The sodium influx is therefore an **electrochemical action**.

Depolarisation and repolarisation

As a result of the sodium influx, the membrane potential moves further away from threshold potential to peak at **+30 mV**, and this is called **depolarisation** (Figure 2.4). As the membrane potential crosses **0 mV**, the membrane changes polarity – that is, the overall negative charge on the *inside* becomes positive, while the overall positive charge on the *outside* becomes negative (Figure 2.4). The inside of the membrane has gained many positive sodium ions and therefore becomes positive, while the outside has lost those same positive sodium ions and therefore becomes negative.

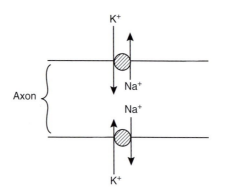

FIGURE 2.5 Sodium–potassium pumps are working during the refractory phase to restore the ions to the original positions; sodium is pumped out of the axon, potassium is pumped in.

At +30 mV (i.e. the peak of an action potential) potassium channels open and allow the rapid movement of potassium out of the axonal membrane. Potassium moves out for the same electrochemical reasons that sodium moved in. The positively charged potassium is attracted to the negative charge outside the membrane and is also flowing down its own concentration gradient, from high inside to low outside. This mass movement of potassium returns the membrane to resting potential, i.e. from +30 mV down to −70 mV again, a process called **repolarisation** (Figure 2.4). As 0 mV is crossed there is another reversal of membrane polarity, from the overall positive inside and negative outside of the action potential, to the overall negative inside and positive outside of the resting potential. However, this restoration of resting potential occurs with the main ions, sodium and potassium, in the reverse positions from when the process started. Before another action potential is possible, the sodium must be returned to the *outside* of the membrane and the potassium returned to the *inside* of the membrane. The membrane has sodium and potassium pumps (Figure 2.5) which pump these ions across the membrane, against their concentration gradients, and thus return the two cations to their former concentrations, sodium outside and potassium inside the axon. The period of time needed for this to take place, and for the sodium and potassium channels to close, is known as the **refractory phase** (Figures 2.4 and 2.5). During this period the axon cannot produce another action potential (Martini 2001).

Figure 2.4 shows the time scale, along the base axis, during which all these events take place. It is significant that the entire action potential occupies between two and three milliseconds (2–3 ms; i.e. two to three thousandths of a second), with a refractory phase lasting another millisecond. Thus, between one action potential and the next there is a time interval of about only four milliseconds, allowing a single neuron a capacity of up to 250 action potentials per second. The speed at which the nervous system works, in thousandths of a second, is faster than the blink of an eye, which to us appears to be instantaneous.

Myelinated and unmyelinated axons

The action potential described also has to pass along the axon from cell to synapse. In an unmyelinated axon, depolarisation at one part of the axonal membrane causes the membrane just ahead to reach threshold and begin the process of depolarisation there. Repeating this process continuously results in a wave of depolarisation that sweeps down the axon. This will be followed by a wave of repolarisation, immediately behind depolarisation, during which resting potential is restored (Figure 2.6). See page 36

In a myelinated axon a different process causes the spread of an action potential down the axon (Figure 2.7). The membrane, which is covered by See page 36

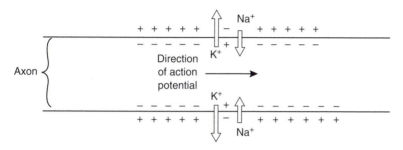

FIGURE 2.6 An unmyelinated axon. The impulse sweeps from left to right, caused by a sodium input, which reverses the membrane charge from resting to action potential, followed right behind by a potassium efflux, which restores the membrane resting potential charge.

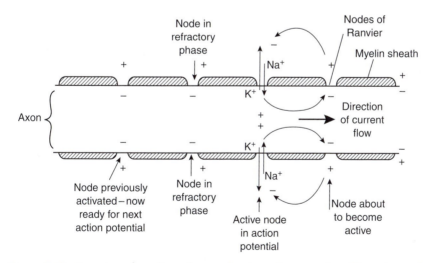

FIGURE 2.7 A section of myelinated axon showing saltatory action. The active node has a sodium influx followed immediately by a potassium efflux – i.e. an action potential. This positive input is attracted to the negative potential on the inside of the next node in the sequence, and this will rapidly reach threshold and action potential. The node behind the active node is in refractory phase.

myelin, cannot allow the passage of ions and so will not be involved in the movement of an action potential. However, the myelination has tiny gaps in it called the **nodes of Ranvier** where depolarisation and repolarisation take place. To describe what is happening, we will take a three-node sequence from a myelinated axon (see Figure 2.7). In Figure 2.7 the active node has reached threshold and will depolarise, i.e. reverse its polarity, while the other nodes are in resting potential. The positive sodium entering at the active node is attracted to the negative on the inside at the next node along and will jump across the myelin internode to reach it. This movement of sodium causes the next node to reach threshold potential and depolarise. While sodium is entering this next node, the previous active node has reached repolarisation with the outflow of potassium. The process of sodium entering at a node and leaping over the internode to the next node is repeated along the length of the axon. This leaping over internodes is called **saltatory** ('jumping') action and speeds up the passage of an action potential down the axon. An action potential can pass along a fully myelinated axon at a speed of up to 120 meters per second compared to 2.3 meters per second along an unmyelinated axon. In either case the speed is fast, with action potentials passing through the full length of the body in a fraction of a second.

Synapses

Synapses (Figure 2.8) are the minute gaps (or **clefts**) occurring between the end of one neuronal axon and the membrane of the structure beyond. The **synaptic cleft**, which is between 20 nm and 50 nm across, separates the **pre-synaptic bulb** from the **postsynaptic membrane**. The presynaptic bulb is an expansion of the axon terminal. Within it there are many vesicles containing a chemical **neurotransmitter** destined to be released into the cleft. Neurotransmitters come in a variety of different forms (see Chapter 3), but

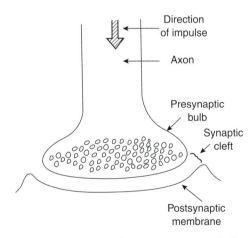

Direction of impulse

Axon

Presynaptic bulb

Synaptic cleft

Postsynaptic membrane

FIGURE 2.8 A synapse. The axon ends in a presynaptic bulb which is filled with vesicles housing a neurotransmitter.

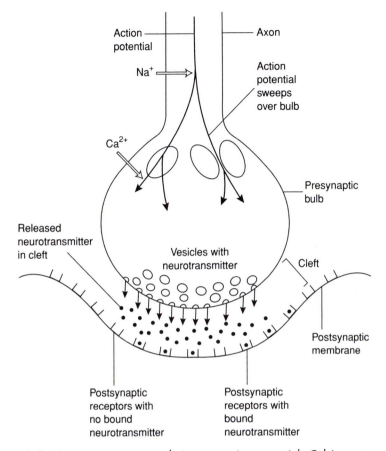

Action
potential

Axon

Na$^+$

Action
potential
sweeps
over bulb

Ca^{2+}

Presynaptic
bulb

Released
neurotransmitter
in cleft

Vesicles with
neurotransmitter

Cleft

Postsynaptic
membrane

Postsynaptic
receptors with
no bound
neurotransmitter

Postsynaptic
receptors with
bound
neurotransmitter

FIGURE 2.9 Events at a synapse during an action potential. Calcium enters the presynaptic bulb and the vesicles flood to the presynaptic membrane; the vesicles rupture and empty their contents into the synaptic cleft. Neurotransmitters can bind to receptors in the postsynaptic membrane and initiate a change in that membrane.

they all have in common the ability to bind to protein receptors attached to the postsynaptic membrane and thus cause a change within that membrane and the cell beyond. This happens when the neurotransmitter is released from the presynaptic bulb in response to the arrival of an action potential (Figure 2.9).

Action potentials sweeping down the axon involve the influx of sodium ions (Na$^+$), but on arrival at the presynaptic bulb the ionic influx changes to a different ion, i.e. the calcium ion (Ca^{2+}). This change to the double positive charge of calcium probably causes an even faster rise to +30 mV in the presynaptic bulb, triggering a sudden migration of the vesicles to the presynaptic membrane. Here they rupture and empty their neuro-transmitter contents into the cleft. These chemicals then flood the cleft and bind to receptor sites on the postsynaptic membrane. The binding of a neurotransmitter, even for only one or two milliseconds, causes important changes in the postsynaptic membrane to which the postsynaptic cell will

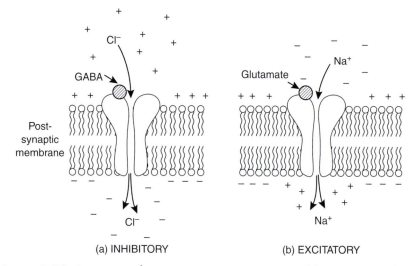

FIGURE 2.10 Two types of postsynaptic receptor. (a) An inhibitory receptor binding GABA (gamma-aminobutyric acid). This causes the opening of a chloride (Cl⁻) channel and chloride enters the postsynaptic membrane. The entry of this negative ion causes the resting potential to become even more negative, preventing any chance of an action potential in that membrane. (b) An excitatory receptor binding glutamate. This causes the opening of a sodium channel and sodium ions (Na⁺) to enter. The entry of a positive ion sets up an action potential in the postsynaptic membrane.

respond. After binding, the neurotransmitters will be removed from the receptor. Some will be broken down and disposed of by excretion via the cerebrospinal fluid (CSF) and the blood to the kidneys. Others are also degraded but reabsorbed back into the presynaptic bulb and recycled. Some neurotransmitters are recycled in part via cells called astrocytes.

See page 35

Excitation and inhibition

Some synapses are **excitatory** in function, while others are **inhibitory** (Figure 2.10). Excitatory synapses cause activity to occur beyond the post-synaptic membrane, often generating an action potential in the membrane of a second neuron. This is achieved by the binding of a neurotrans-mitter to receptors of the postsynaptic membrane which are linked to sodium channels in that membrane. The neurotransmitter causes the recep-tor to open the sodium channel; sodium then floods into the membrane from its high concentration outside the membrane, and starts a new action potential.

Inhibitory synapses do the opposite. The receptor is linked to a chloride (Cl⁻) channel which is opened by the binding of neurotransmitter allowing chloride to enter the postsynaptic membrane. Chloride will move down its concentration gradient from the higher concentrations found outside the membrane (Figure 2.3). The resting potential of that membrane, i.e. negative on the inside, becomes even more negative, ensuring that any action potentials in that neuron are impossible (i.e. they are inhibited). At first sight this may seem surprising. After all, the nervous system is designed to generate action potentials, so the blocking (or inhibition) of action potentials appears to go against the very purpose of the system. However, think for a moment about the motor car. It is designed to move (a car that does not move is a waste of time), yet one of the fundamental components is a braking system, designed to prevent any movement. Is that surprising? Of course not, since a car that cannot stop is deadly. And so it is with the brain. Uncontrolled, unchecked action potentials would be like a car going downhill with no brakes. Life for the person with no inhibitory synapses would be a living nightmare. Every action potential would cause some form of activity; there would never be any rest, day or night, for the brain or the body. Compare the inhibitory synapses with the 'off' switch on a computer, where activation causes a shut-down of the system. Every system, including the nervous system, needs a form of deactivation at some point.

Neuromodulators

Neurotransmitters and their receptor binding sites are critical, not only to the function of the entire nervous system but also to the mechanism of action of many psychotropic drugs, and therefore a more detailed discussion of these chemicals and their receptors is given in Chapter 3. However, in addition to neurotransmitters, chemicals called neuromodulators are also produced at the synapse. The term **neuromodulator** can be applied to various substances which are often released along with a neurotransmitter. These neuromodulators have a generally wider effect on neuronal function than neurotransmitters for the following reasons:

1 Neurotransmitters are released in small quantities and act locally within the synapse in which they are released. Neuromodulators are released in larger quantities and spread out beyond the synapse from which they are released. They therefore influence many other synaptic connections over a larger area of the brain.
2 Neuromodulators appear to modify the response of receptors to the neurotransmitter.
3 Some neuromodulators may act by binding to autoreceptors, which are receptors situated on the presynaptic membrane of the bulb, thus modifying the release of neurotransmitters (Rosenzweig *et al.* 1999).

Neuromodulators are mostly **neuropeptides**, i.e. small proteins of the nervous system. However, several substances usually classified as neurotransmitters may have a neuromodulatory role by acting beyond the synapse from where they were released, e.g. **enkephalin** and **choleceystokinin** (see Chapter 3). Several groups of **hormones** are also peptides. Hormones have an even *See page 63* wider influence over the activity of the brain (as well as the body) by being released into the blood circulation. Hormonal influence over brain activity is discussed in Chapter 5.

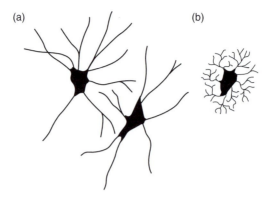

FIGURE 2.11 Astrocytes: (a) fibrous; (b) protoplasmic.

Neuroglia

Astrocytes

Neuroglia, or glial cells, are the support cells of the central nervous system. They outnumber the neurons by nine to one (there are 900 billion neuroglia compared with 100 billion neurons), but they do not create or transmit action potentials (impulses) as neurons do. Of this vast number, the commonest glial cells are the **astrocytes** (Figure 2.11), so called because of their star shape, created by many fine extensions pushing out in all directions. There are two forms of astrocyte; the **fibrous** form and the **protoplasmic** form. The fibrous form is largely found in the white matter of the brain. Fibrous astrocytes have fewer processes than their protoplasmic cousins, but their processes are long and straight, some with broad ends (like feet), which attach to blood capillaries or to the cells of the pia mater. The fibrous astrocytes respond to brain tissue injury by growing in large numbers (a process called **gliosis**). Unlike most neurons, both kinds of astrocyte retain the ability to go through mitosis (cell division) for the duration of the person's lifetime. The protoplasmic forms appear mostly in the grey matter of the brain. Their processes are shorter but more numerous than in the fibrous type, each process being more extensively branched.

See page 3

Astrocytes generally have a very close association with neurons, surrounding the cell bodies and synapses, as well as blood capillaries, with their processes. The function of astrocytes is only now beginning to come to light (Bear *et al.* 1996). They appear to have a role to play during the moment when neurons are transmitting an action potential. Neuronal action potentials cause the adjacent astrocytes to increase their metabolism and at the same time to partly depolarise, although they do not themselves achieve an action potential. Potassium ions (K^+) flood out from the axonal membrane of the neuron as the action potential sweeps down towards the synapse, and the astrocyte takes up this extracellular potassium in order to stabilise the ionic environment around the neuron. Excess *extracellular* potassium is dangerous to the brain and, if it got into circulation, it would

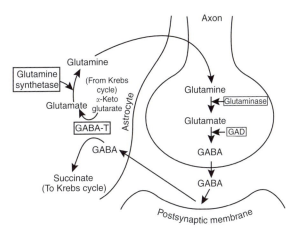

FIGURE 2.12 Astrocytes near a GABA synapse are partly involved in the GABA–glutamate synthesis cycle. The enzymes are in boxes: GABA-T = gamma-aminobutyric acid transaminase; GAD = glutamic acid decarboxylase.

be dangerous to the heart. Potassium is normally kept concentrated *inside* the cells.

Astrocytes are also involved in the biochemistry of neurotransmitters. They are often found surrounding the synapse, where they prevent neurotransmitter leakage and assist in the removal and, in some cases, the recycling of neurotransmitters after these chemicals have fulfilled their task. One such form of neurotransmitter recycling that involves the astrocyte is the production of glutamate from gamma-aminobutyric acid (GABA) within the cytoplasm of an astrocyte close to the GABA synapse. The glutamate thus created is passed back from the astrocyte to the neuron for the further synthesis of GABA (Figure 2.12), a good example of the supportive role of these cells.

Some astrocytes have been found to bind neurotransmitters to receptor sites attached to the astrocyte membrane, although the purpose of binding of neurotransmitters to astrocytes is not fully known (Bear *et al.* 1996). In one example of this, glutamate, an important neurotransmitter of several brain areas such as the cerebrum, was added to astrocytes. On binding to receptor sites it caused the astrocyte to oscillate between high and low calcium levels within its cytoplasm. These calcium waves within the cell have been seen to pass on to other cells through membrane-to-membrane contacts between adjacent astrocytes. In one experiment, a calcium wave induced in one astrocyte by adding glutamate was witnessed to pass through 59 other attached astrocytes before it stopped. Such calcium surges must indicate a form of cell signalling about which much is still to be learnt (Young 1997). Other functions of astrocytes have been proposed from varying amounts of evidence. For example, the broad feet resting on blood capillaries suggest a possible nutritional role for these cells. It would not be possible for every one of 100 billion neurons to receive its own blood supply. Many neurons rely on nutrients being collected from the circulation by astrocytes and passed on to the neurons, with wastes possibly going in

35

the opposite direction. Astrocytes also store glucose and pass this on to the neurons for energy purposes.

The importance of studying astrocytes is highlighted in this list of functions. Gliosis (excessive growth of glial cells) is somehow involved in brain repair, and this mechanism may have implications for mental health, such as in dementia. Also, the role of astrocytes in neurotransmitter recycling could be of importance in depression or anxiety, and the fact that they have neurotransmitter receptors now makes them possible targets for psychotropic drugs. Such future drugs may be used to modify mental activity by affecting astrocytes, with or without neuronal involvement, and it is possible that some current drugs may already be influencing mental activity through astrocyte involvement.

Other glial cells

The glial cells that form myelin sheaths around axons fall into two types, the **oligodendrocytes** within the central nervous system only, and the **Schwann cells** within the peripheral nervous system only. Myelination, as identified earlier, is essential for the saltatory passage of action potentials. Some neurons remain unmyelinated but they are less numerous. Oligodendrocytes are small cells within the brain and cord, and during embryonic development each cell contributes myelination to several axons at once. Each Schwann cell, however, contributes myelination to only one segment of a single peripheral axon (Figure 2.1). Both types of cell leave gaps (the nodes of Ranvier) between the myelination patches where short sections of axon are exposed (Figure 2.1).

Glial cells include the following other types:

- The **microglia**, small phagocytic cells of the central nervous system (CNS, i.e. the brain and spinal cord), which engulf and remove not only invading organisms but also remnants and debris of dead cells.
- The **ependymal cells**, flat cells lining the brain's ventricular system and ducts, which provide a smooth surface for the cerebrospinal fluid (CSF) to flow over. They have cilia (minute hair-like processes) on the cell surface which produce a sweeping action that aids the circulation of CSF.
- The **satellite cells**, the smallest cells of the brain, associated with neuronal cell bodies and Schwann cells, whose function is not yet known.

Ependymal cells fall into three main groups. The **ependymocytes** line the ventricles and central canal of the spinal cord. The **tanycytes** line the floor of the third ventricle and have processes touching blood capillaries; they may be involved in the movement of hormones from the blood to the adjacent hypothalamus. The **choroidal cells** cover the choroid plexus and promote the production of CSF.

During embryonic development of the nervous system, ependymal cells take on another role related to the migration of neurons within the neural tube (the embryonic stage of development of the central nervous system).

They form a temporary framework along which the migrating neuron will move from its site of cellular mitosis. This framework is rather like a trellis along which a plant will grow. The process of neuronal migration is important for the correct location of neurons in the brain and the establishment of their subsequent synaptic connections. If the wrong route is taken by neurons along the ependymal framework, inappropriate synaptic connections will be formed. This malformation is implicated in several mental health disorders, notably schizophrenia, and is discussed further in Chapter 8.

Key points

The neuron

- Neurons are the functional unit of the nervous system. They have a cell body bearing dendrites and an axon.
- Axons are efferent pathways conveying action potentials to the synapse. They are mostly myelinated to speed up the passage of action potentials.
- Axonal transportation allows for the passage of proteins and some neurotransmitters from the cell body, down the axon to the synapse.

Neurotransmission

- The membrane begins in resting potential, with sodium concentrated outside the axon and potassium concentrated inside the axon.
- Action potentials are generated by a sodium influx into the axon, followed by a potassium output from the axon, which restores resting potential.

Synapses

- Synapses store neurotransmitters, which are released into the cleft on arrival of the action potential. Neurotransmitters then bind to the postsynaptic membrane and cause changes beyond that membrane.
- Synapses are either excitatory (causing changes such as action potentials in the postsynaptic membrane) or inhibitory (blocking such changes).
- Neuromodulators are neuropeptides produced at the synapse.
- Neuromodulators have a wide effect on neuronal function by spreading out beyond the synapse they are released from.
- Neuromodulators may modify the response of receptors to the neurotransmitter and help to control the release of neurotransmitters.

Neuroglia

- Neuroglia are the support cells of the nervous system. Astrocytes are the most numerous of the neuroglia, providing nutritional, ionic and neurotransmitter support to neurons.
- Oligodendrocytes (within the brain and cord) and Schwann cells (within the peripheral nerves) provide myelination to axons.

References

Bear M. F., Connors B. W. and Paradiso M. A. (1996) *Neuroscience, Exploring the Brain*, Williams and Wilkins, Baltimore.

Blows W. T. (2000) Systems and diseases: The nervous system 1. *Nursing Times*, **96** (35): 41–44.

Blows W. T. (2001) *The Biological Basis of Nursing: Clinical Observations*. Routledge, London.

Day M. (1997) Brain cells defy division rule. *New Scientist*, 19 April.

Martini F. H. (2001) *Anatomy and Physiology* (5th edn). Prentice Hall, Upper Saddle River, NJ.

Rosenzweig M. R., Leiman A. L. and Breedlove S. M. (1999) *Biological Psychology, An Introduction to Behavioural, Cognitive and Clinical Neuroscience* (2nd edn). Sinauer Associates, Sunderland, MA.

Young S. (1997) Brain cells hit the big time. *New Scientist Planet Science* http://www.newscientist.com/ns/970531/nlead2.html

Chapter 3

Neurotransmitters and receptors

- Introduction to neurotransmitters
- Receptors
- The amine neurotransmitters
- The amino acid neurotransmitters
- The peptide neurotransmitters
- Endogenous opioids
- Other neurotransmitters
- Key points

Introduction to neurotransmitters

Neurotransmitters are the chemical agents released from the presynaptic bulb into the synaptic cleft. They are sometimes referred to as the *primary messenger*, since they occur as free chemicals that move across a space (here it is the cleft) and cause a change in another part (in this case, the postsynaptic membrane). Another term used for neurotransmitters is **ligand**, meaning an agent that binds to a receptor and in so doing changes that receptor. The main change that occurs in receptors on binding of a ligand is an **allosteric** effect, i.e. a change of receptor *shape*. This change then has a further effect, the nature of which depends on which receptor is considered; it may be either within the membrane or beyond it in the cytoplasm of the cell.

Most neurotransmitters fall into three main groups, the **amines**, the **amino acids** and the **peptides**. Amines are compounds containing the **amino group** (NH_2) and amines have the general structure RCH_2NH_2 where R is a variable portion (known as a **radical**) (Figure 3.1a). Variations in the radical give

39

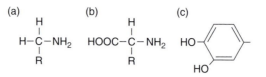

FIGURE 3.1 The structure of three compounds: (a) an amine; (b) an amino acid; (c) the catechol group. NH_2 is the amino group; COOH is the carboxyl group; R is the radical (variable portion).

rise to different amines. Amino acids, the building blocks of proteins, are amines in which a **carboxyl group** (**COOH**) replaces one of the hydrogens on a carbon atom (Figure 3.1b). A peptide is a small protein, i.e. a small number of amino acids bonded together in a linear chain. Acetylcholine is a neurotransmitter of different origin and is discussed separately. **Catecholamines** are amines combined with a **catechol group** (Figure 3.1c), which consists of a carbon ring with two OH branches. A discussion related to each of the better-known neurotransmitters follows, as this information is relevant to an understanding of the neuropathology of the various mental health disorders and to neuropharmacology.

See page 58

See page 43

Receptors

Specific activity at the synapse is not due to the function of any particular neurotransmitter but to the function of the receptor to which it binds. By binding to different receptors, the *same* neurotransmitter is often seen to produce *different* effects. Receptors for any given neurotransmitter fall into several types (or groups) according to structure and function, and each receptor type usually has distinct subtypes. A good example is acetylcholine, which binds to two main types of receptors, either nicotinic or muscarinic, and these have subtypes (e.g. muscarinic subtypes are M_1, M_2, M_3, M_4, M_5). Subtle variations in the way these subtypes respond to acetylcholine binding result in a wide range of activity for the neurotransmitter.

It is also important to recognise two other ways of classifying receptor sites:

1 According to their *location*. **Postsynaptic receptors** are part of the *postsynaptic* membrane of the cell that occurs beyond the cleft. Their purpose, when activated by neurotransmitter, is to effect some kind of change within that postsynaptic cell, such as the generation of a new action potential. Alternatively, **autoreceptors** are found on some *presynaptic* membranes or other parts of the neuron and therefore allow neurotransmitters to bind to the same neuron that releases it. Such autoreceptors are thought to provide feedback information to the neuron and the presynaptic bulb, in particular, to regulate (or control) any further neurotransmitter release (Bear *et al.* 1996).
2 According to their *function*. Some receptors are **ionotropic**. They control the opening or closing of a particular ion channel and can do this remarkably quickly, usually within milliseconds. When a neurotransmitter

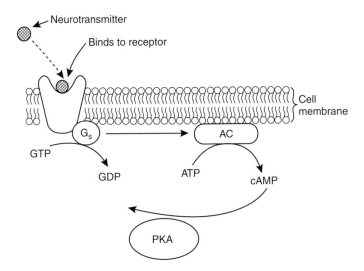

FIGURE 3.2 An excitatory metabotropic receptor. The neurotransmitter (first messenger) binds to the receptor outside the membrane. This activates a stimulatory G-protein (G$_s$), which binds guanosine triphosphate (GTP) and forms guanosine diphosphate (GDP). The activated G$_s$ protein moves along the inner membrane, and collides with and activates adenylyl cyclase (AC). This in turn binds adenosine triphosphate (ATP) to form cyclic adenosine monophosphate (cAMP). cAMP is free to move into the cell (it is a second messenger) and activate protein kinase A (PKA), which can have a multitude of different effects on the cell. Compare with Figure 3.3.

binds to a receptor, the receptor changes shape (the allosteric effect) and this opens a channel in the membrane, e.g. a sodium channel, allowing ions to pass through the membrane. The passage of sodium ions (positively charged cations) into a second neuron will initiate a new action potential and therefore occurs at **excitatory** synapses (Figure 2.10). The passage of chloride (a negatively charged anion) into a second neuron will prevent an action potential and therefore occurs at **inhibitory** synapses (Figure 2.10).

Other receptors are **metabotropic** (Figure 3.2). They do not *directly* influence ionic channels but do cause changes in the metabolism of the postsynaptic cell.

The binding of a neurotransmitter to metabotropic receptors causes activation of a membrane-bound protein on the inside of the cell. This is the **G-protein**, abbreviated from *guanosine triphosphate (GTP) binding protein*, which may have an inhibitory (**G$_i$**) or a stimulatory (**G$_s$**) effect on cellular enzymes. In this way, metabotropic receptors, like ionotropic receptors, can also be excitatory or inhibitory. However, because they operate through a different mechanism, they are slower than ionotropic receptors and their effects remain over a longer period of time. When the G$_s$ protein is activated, it moves along the inside of the membrane until it contacts a membrane-bound enzyme called **adenylyl cyclase** (**AC**). Allosteric activation of AC then occurs and this enzyme binds and splits intracellular ATP to form

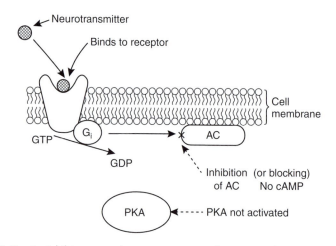

FIGURE 3.3 An inhibitory metabotropic receptor. The activated inhibitory G_i protein collides with adenylyl cyclase (AC), which is then deactivated and unable to form cyclic adenosine monophosphate (cAMP). As a result, protein kinase A (PKA) is not activated. Compare with Figure 3.2.

cAMP (cyclic adenosine monophosphate). cAMP is known as a **secondary messenger** because it is free to move through the cell (unlike the G_s protein and AC which are bound to the inside of the postsynaptic membrane). The primary messenger was the neurotransmitter, which was free to move around the synaptic cleft. The secondary messenger is free to move around the inside of the cell (the **cytosol**). Secondary messengers like cAMP, or others such as **inositol trisphosphate** (**IP₃**) and **diacylglycerol** (**DAG**) produced by some metabotropic receptors, then go on to influence other cellular functions. IP₃ opens calcium channels, whilst cAMP and DAG activate an enzyme known as **protein kinase** (**PK**). When activated, PK regulates changes in the cell's metabolism. This may involve the opening of ion channels, causing changes in the ionic environment of the cell, the moderation of protein synthesis, or even the activation of specific genes leading to protein synthesis (**gene expression**) (Figure 3.2). Metabotropic receptors that activate G_i proteins are inhibitory because they block any activity of AC (Figure 3.3).

Receptors are actually proteins set into the cell membrane and they have a specific role which is activated by the binding of neurotransmitter. Some receptors are attached to the outer surface of the membrane, while others are transmembranous (i.e. they pass right through the membrane, appearing on both sides). Cells can of course produce proteins, so they can also produce receptors when necessary. This means that cells can **upregulate** their receptors by producing more of them, increasing the receptor density of their membrane and therefore binding more of the neurotransmitter. This is likely to be the consequence of reduced quantities of available neurotransmitter.

Alternatively, cells can **downregulate** their membrane receptor density by slowing receptor production, especially if the neurotransmitter is in

abundance. Measurements of receptor density on postsynaptic membranes give useful information about the levels of neurotransmitter present
in the synaptic cleft. This is important because variations in the level of
neurotransmitter can affect mental health, causing, for example, depression
(Nemeroff 1998).

See page 184

We will now move on to consider some of the major neurotransmitters
and their receptors, and, where it is understood, their role in maintaining
mental health.

The amine neurotransmitters

Dopamine

Dopamine, noradrenaline and adrenaline are three **catecholamine** neurotransmitters that share a common pathway of production (Figure 3.4). The
starting point for the production of dopamine is the dietary amino acid
tyrosine, which is converted by the neurons to **dihydroxyphenylalanine**
(known as **dopa**) by the enzyme **tyrosine hydroxylase**. Further convertion
to dopamine is by another enzyme called **dopa decarboxylase**. After use,
dopamine is broken down in two sites, within the cleft and in the presynaptic
bulb, by several enzymes including one called **monoamine oxidase** (**MAO**)
which is situated at the junction of the axon with the bulb. The final metabolite, **homovanillic acid**, is excreted via the CSF.

See page 196
See page 171

Dopamine activates several important pathways of the brain (Figure 3.5).
From the brain stem nucleus known as the **ventral tegmental area** (**VTA**),
closely associated with the substantia nigra, two major dopaminergic (i.e.

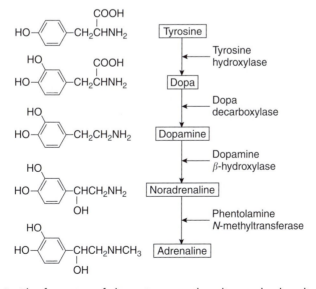

FIGURE 3.4 The formation of dopamine, noradrenaline and adrenaline from the
amino acid tyrosine. The products are boxed, while the enzymes (unboxed) label the
arrows. The chemical structure of each product is shown on the left.

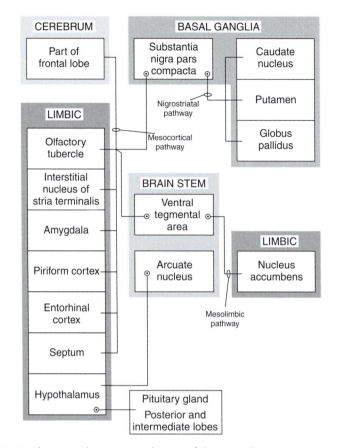

FIGURE 3.5 The main dopamine pathways of the central nervous system.

responding to dopamine) tracts pass out to specific brain areas. One tract passes to the **cerebral cortex**, forming the **mesocortical pathway**, and the other to the **nucleus accumbens** of the **limbic system**, forming the **mesolimbic pathway**. An additional major dopaminergic pathway is the tract from the **substantia nigra** in the midbrain to other main areas of the **basal ganglia**, forming the **nigrostriatal pathway**. Some authors join the nigrostriatal and mesolimbic pathways together under the term **mesostriatal system**.

In some sites of the brain, dopamine acts as an inhibitory neurotransmitter, although, as discussed, the function of a neurotransmitters more often relates to the receptor that it binds to than to the ligand itself. In this capacity, dopamine is involved in inhibiting muscle tone, a function of the substantia nigra (see Parkinson's disease). It also inhibits breast milk production by blocking the release of the hormone **prolactin** from the anterior **pituitary gland** when the woman is not breast-feeding. Dopamine also plays a vital role in the function of the limbic system and here it is associated with brain arousal. It is implicated in psychotic disturbances such as hallucinations in schizophrenia and manic-depressive

See page 40

See page 224

See page 170

psychosis, as well as being involved in the reward pathways associated with drug addiction (Blows 2000). *See page 114*

Dopamine receptors

Dopamine receptors are all metabotropic. Five subclasses of dopamine receptor are identified (D_1, D_2, D_3, D_4 and D_5). D_1 is excitatory and increases the level of cAMP in the cell, whilst D_2 is either inhibitory and reduces the activity of cAMP or does not affect it. The D_3 receptor is found in the limbic system and in particular the hypothalamus, while D_4 is mostly found in the cortex, hippocampus, amygdala and nucleus accumbens. The specific functions of D_4 and D_5 are as yet unknown.

Noradrenaline

Noradrenaline (norepinephrine) is produced from dopamine by the action of the enzyme **dopamine β-hydroxylase** (**DBH**) (Figure 3.4). Noradrenaline is produced both as a hormone from the **adrenal medulla** as well as a neurotransmitter in parts of the brain and at the **sympathetic** nerve terminals. *See page 16* The adrenergic (responding to noradrenaline) brain pathways centre primarily on the **locus coeruleus** in the brain stem. Tracts from this nucleus pass out to the cerebrum and limbic system (Figure 3.6) as part of the **diffuse modulatory systems** similar to serotonin pathways (see serotonin) (Blows 2000). *See pages 46, 184*

Adrenaline

Adrenaline (epinephrine) is the final stage in the production of catecholamine transmitters. Noradrenaline is acted on by the enzyme **phentolamine *N*-methyltransferase** (**PNMT**) to produce adrenaline (Figure 3.4).

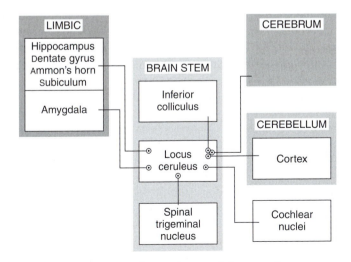

FIGURE 3.6 The main noradrenaline pathways of the central nervous system.

Adrenaline is well known as a *hormone* of the **adrenal medulla**, but as a *neurotransmitter* it is far less well understood. This is because it is found in low concentrations across many widespread sites in the brain. It does not usually occur in specific nuclei, and this pattern of diffuse distribution makes it difficult to study, resulting in a poor understanding of its role in the brain.

Adrenergic receptors

Adrenergic receptors, i.e. those that bind and respond to noradrenaline and adrenaline, are either alpha (α) or beta (β), with subtypes of each (α_1, α_2, β_1, β_2, β_3). They are all metabotropic, activating cellular changes through secondary messengers. The α_1 type is excitatory, and the activation of this receptor causes depolarisation by releasing calcium stored inside the cell. This receptor is found in the brain as a postsynaptic receptor and also in the vascular and intestinal smooth muscle and the heart. The α_2 type is inhibitory (i.e. it uses a G_i protein) and deactivates calcium channels, thus having the opposite effect to α_1 receptors. α_2 receptors are found in the brain as autoreceptors as well as postsynaptic receptors. They are also located in the same smooth muscles as α_1 and on the surface of platelets and nerve terminals.

Beta receptors, on activation by noradrenaline, increase the postsynaptic membrane response to other excitatory stimuli by indirectly affecting ion channels via a series of intermediate proteins which increase cAMP. Both β_1 and β_2 are found in the brain, whilst the β_3 type is located in adipose tissue.

Serotonin

See page 184

Serotonin, an important neurotransmitter, is part of the brain's **diffuse modulatory systems**. Nine nuclei (the **raphe nuclei**) in the brain stem send out serotonergic (responding to serotonin) pathways to many parts of the cerebrum and limbic system (Figure 3.7). The serotonergic system has influence over a wide range of brain functions including regulation of mood, movement, appetite, sexual activity, sleeping and some glandular secretions (Blows 2000). It therefore plays a vital role in the maintenance of mental health and will be discussed again when considering a number of conditions, such as depression and eating disorders.

Serotonin is also known as **5-hydroxytryptamine (5-HT)** and is originally derived from the dietary amino acid **tryptophan**. This crosses the **blood–brain barrier** into the brain, transported by a molecule called the **large neutral amino acid transporter (LNAA)**. The blood–brain barrier is a layer of cells between the circulating blood and the brain tissue and acts like a filter, allowing some molecules to pass into the brain but not others. Since LNAA transports several amino acids into the brain, particularly tyrosine, valine and leucine, the amount of tryptophan entering the brain is dependent on its concentration compared with the concentration of the other amino acids involved. Neurons that use serotonin have the enzyme

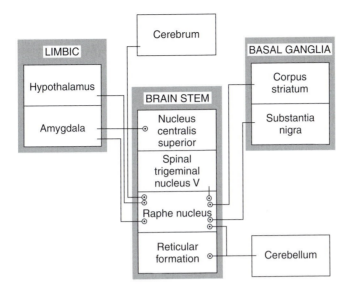

FIGURE 3.7 The main serotonin pathways of the central nervous system.

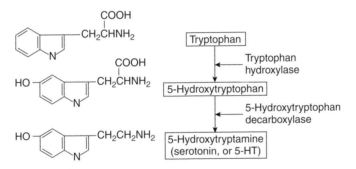

FIGURE 3.8 The formation of serotonin (5-hydroxytryptamine, or 5-HT) from the amino acid tryptophan. The products are boxed while the enzymes (unboxed) label the arrows. The chemical structure of each product is shown on the left.

tryptophan hydroxylase (**TRPH**) in order to convert tryptophan to **5-hydroxytryptophan**, and this is further converted to serotonin by a second enzyme known as **aromatic amino acid decarboxylase (AAAD)**. **Vitamin B$_6$ (pyridoxine)** is vital in the function of AAAD, and thus is important overall in the production of serotonin (Figure 3.8). After its release into the synaptic cleft and after it has bound to postsynaptic receptors, serotonin is taken back into the presynaptic bulb (a process called re-uptake) and broken down. The enzymes that are responsible for this breakdown are monoamine oxidase (MAO) and **aldehyde oxidase**, resulting in a **metabolite** (or waste product) called **5-hydroxyindoleacetic acid (5-HIAA)**. This is excreted first via the cerebrospinal fluid, then to the blood that carries it to the kidneys.

TABLE 3.1 Classes of serotonin receptors and their intracellular actions

Serotonin receptor class	Receptor subclasses	Intracellular role
5-HT1	5-HT1A, 1B, 1D, 1E	Different effects, some reduce AC activity
5-HT2	5-HT2A, 2B, 2C	Activates DAG and IP$_3$
5-HT3		Opens Ca^{2+} channels
5-HT4		Increases cAMP
5-HT5	5-HT5A, 5B	
5-HT6		Increases cAMP
5-HT7		Increases cAMP

Serotonin receptors

Serotonin receptors form many classes and subclasses, all of which are metabotropic. Table 3.1 shows the main classes and subclasses and their intracellular action on binding serotonin, where fully known.

The amino acid neurotransmitters

Glutamate and GABA

Glutamate and **gamma-aminobutyric acid (GABA)** are important neurotransmitters found throughout the cerebral cortex and they share a common synthesis pathway (Figure 3.9, and see also Figure 2.12). Glutamate (glutamic acid) is a potent excitatory transmitter involved in consciousness. It is produced mostly during the daytime as a result of cerebral activity. The synthesis of glutamate is linked with the **tricarboxylic acid** (or **Krebs**) **cycle**, the energy cycle of the neuron. **α-Ketoglutarate**, a component of this cycle, is converted to glutamate by the enzyme **GABA transaminase (GABA-T)**. After use, glutamate is acted on by a second enzyme called **glutamic acid decarboxylase (GAD)** to produce GABA (Figure 3.9).

GABA is a major inhibitory neurotransmitter. After use it is converted to **succinate** by GABA-T (the same enzyme that acted on α-ketoglutarate). Succinate becomes another component of the tricarboxylic cycle. Both enzymes, GABA-T and GAD, rely on a co-factor called **pyridoxal phosphate (PLP)** in order to function. PLP itself relies on a supply of **pyroxidine (vitamin B6)**, and thus glutamate and GABA are both indirectly dependent on vitamin B$_6$ in the diet. GABA-T is most active in astrocytes located close to GABA synapses, while GAD is active in the presynaptic bulb of glutamate neurons (see Figure 2.12). The major glutamate pathways of the brain are shown in Figure 3.10 and the major GABA pathways in Figure 3.11.

Glutamate receptors

The term 'glutamate receptors' is used for those receptors that bind glutamate, but in reality other excitatory amino acids, such as aspartate, can also bind to

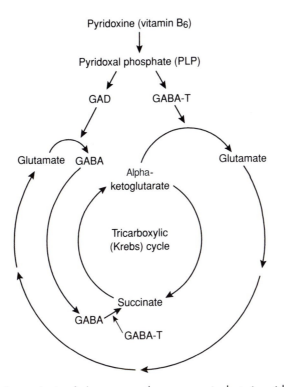

Figure 3.9 The synthesis of glutamate and gamma-aminobutyric acid (GABA). The two main enzymes involved are gamma-aminobutyric acid transaminase (GABA-T) and glutamic acid decarboxylase (GAD). Notice that vitamin B$_6$ is required to form pyridoxal phosphate (PLP), which is essential for both enzymes. Note also the involvement of the tricarboxylic (Krebs) cycle.

and activate the same receptors. ***Glutamate (excitatory amino acid) receptors*** occur in seven known different classes (Carlson 2001), but only five classes are currently well understood. Each of these five is named after the artificial substance that is used as a ligand to bind to it in laboratory conditions. They are mostly ionotropic excitatory receptors with the exception of AMPA (see below), and are linked to ion channels which, when open, allow the passage of positive ions, causing action potentials in the postsynaptic membrane.

The **AMPA (α-amino-3-hydroxy-5-methyl-4-isoxazoleproprionate)** receptors are the most common type of receptor found in the brain. There are two subtypes, one being metabotropic (sometimes classified separately as the **metabotropic glutamate receptor**) (Carlson 2001) and the other ionotropic. The ionotropic receptor is not specific to any particular positive ion.

The **K (kainic acid)** receptor is a nonspecific ion channel receptor causing depolarisation in the cell when activated.

The **NMDA (*N*-methyl-*D*-aspartate)** receptor (Figure 3.12) is the most potent and best-understood of the excitatory amino acid receptors. It is mostly in the cerebral cortex, especially in areas concerned with learning

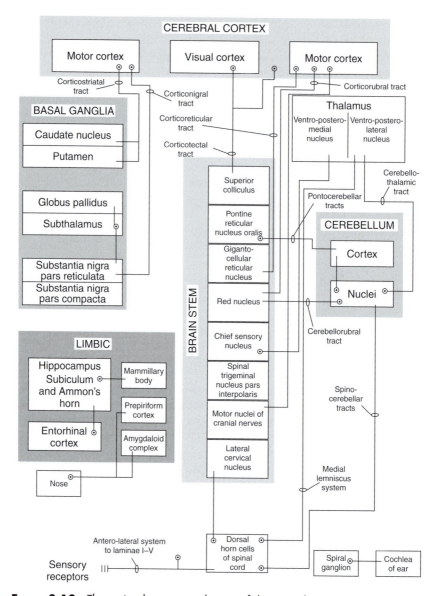

FIGURE 3.10 The main glutamate pathways of the central nervous system.

See page 242 and memory, such as the hippocampus. When inactivated, the ion channel that forms part of the receptor is both closed and blocked by a magnesium (Mg^{2+}) plug on its inner surface. Activation of the receptor requires the binding of both glutamate and glycine, which together cause allosteric changes that open the channel. Removal of the Mg^{2+} plug is achieved by voltage changes across the membrane, occurring when AMPA or K channels are opened farther along on the same membrane. In this way, NMDA receptors function in harmony with other excitatory amino acid receptors. Calcium movement through the open channel causes the biggest

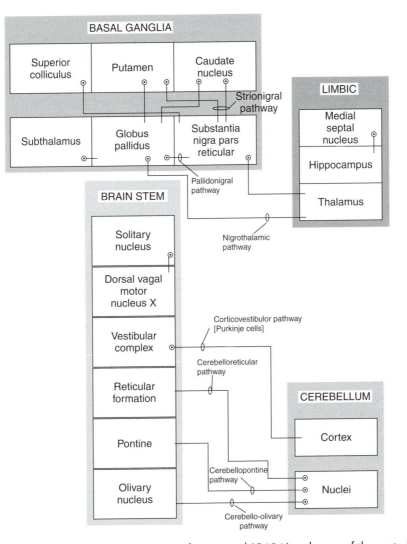

FIGURE 3.11 The main gamma-aminobutyric acid (GABA) pathways of the central nervous system.

depolarisation, with sodium and potassium movements also occurring (Figure 3.12).

The **ACPD** and the **LAP4** receptors, like the NMDA receptor, also cause excitation of the neuron by increasing the volume of intracellular calcium. Unlike NMDA, ACPD and LAP4 activation causes the release of calcium already stored within the cell in the endoplasmic reticulum.

GABA receptors

GABA receptors are of two subtypes, $GABA_A$ and $GABA_B$. The $GABA_A$ receptor (Figure 3.13) is ionotropic, where GABA opens a chloride channel

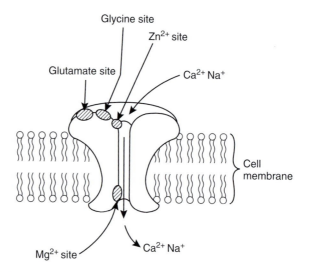

FIGURE 3.12 The NMDA glutamate receptor. Ca^{2+} is the calcium ion, Na^+ is the sodium ion, Mg^{2+} is the magnesium ion and Zn^{2+} is the zinc ion.

in the postsynaptic membrane. When chloride (Cl^-) enters the cell, it hyperpolarises the membrane and therefore prevents action potentials (Figure 3.13). By blocking action potentials in this way, GABA is said to be inhibitory, and therefore reduces the overall activity of the brain. The $GABA_A$ receptor is the site of binding for several important drugs used in psychiatry, the benzodiazipines and the barbiturates, as well as binding alcohol.

See page 155
See page 128

The $GABA_B$ receptor is metabotropic, causing reduced AC activity and reduced levels of intracellular calcium.

Aspartate and glycine

Aspartate (Figure 3.14) and **glycine** are two nonessential amino acid neurotransmitters and neurons can synthesise them as required (i.e. they are not directly obtained from the diet). Aspartate is, like glutamate, another excitatory neurotransmitter. Although aspartate is widely distributed throughout the brain, aspartate concentrations are generally weaker than those of glutamate, except in the ventral motor pathways of the cord. Glycine is, like GABA, another mostly inhibitory neurotransmitter. The distribution of glycine in the central nervous system is similar to that of aspartate, being less widely distributed than GABA and somewhat less well concentrated in spinal motor neurons than aspartate.

The peptide neurotransmitters

Generally, peptide neurotransmitters are produced from **precursors** – that is, protein gene products from which the final neuropeptide is obtained by enzymic action. These peptides are often found in both the digestive tract

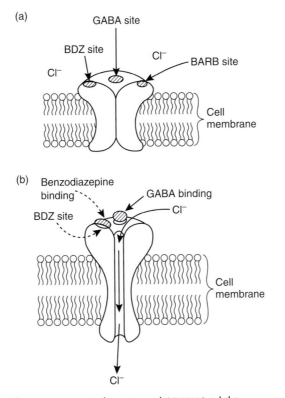

Figure 3.13 The gamma-aminobutyric acid (GABA) inhibitory receptor (GABA_A). (a) The closed receptor with no GABA binding. Notice the BDZ (benzodiazepine) and the BARB (barbiturate) binding sites. (b) The open receptor with GABA and benzodiazepine binding. The opening through the cell membrane is a chloride (Cl⁻) channel.

and the brain. In the brain they appear to be concentrated mostly in the hypothalamus. The hypothalamus is known for many functions, one of which is the control of appetite.

See page 10

Cholecystokinin

Cholecystokinin (CCK) is a peptide found both in the digestive tract (where is regulates emptying of the gall bladder) and in the brain. It is derived from the precursor **procholecystokinin**, which is found in the cerebral cortex and the hypothalamus. A number of different cholecystokinins are produced from this precursor, the best ones studied in the brain being CCK4 and CCK8 (Wild and Benzel 1994). Cholecystokinin in the hypothalamus is involved in regulating the inhibition of food intake once the stomach is full (a process called **satiation**), controlled by the **satiety centre** of the hypothalamus. The function of cholecystokinin in the cerebral cortex is unknown. CCK8 is also concentrated in the hippocampus, amygdala and the spinal cord. It is often

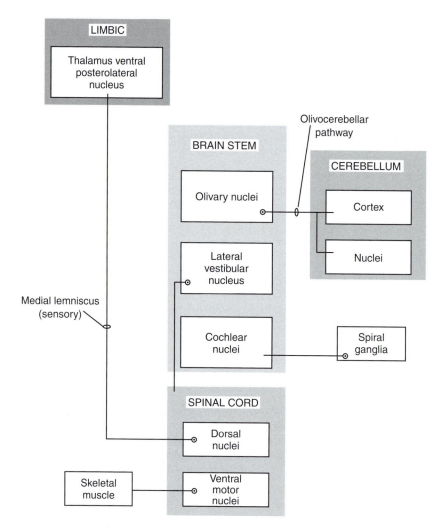

FIGURE 3.14 The main aspartate pathways of the central nervous system.

found associated with dopaminergic neurons, notably in the nigrostrial pathway and the nucleus accumbens, and must have a function related to the role of dopamine.

Neuropeptide Y

Neuropeptide Y (NPY) is a neurotransmitter known to occur in pathways connecting the **arcuate nucleus** (part of the basal **hypothalamus**) to the lateral hypothalamus. Release of neuropeptide Y causes an increase in eating, the neurotransmitter itself being a powerful stimulator of food intake. There are two groups of neurons in the lateral hypothalamus activated by NPY: those that secrete **melanin-concentrating hormone (MCH)** and those that secrete **orexin**, both of which are peptides that stimulate appetite and lower body metabolism. Since NPY has some control over normal food intake, disturbance of NPY may be related to some eating disorders. *See page 152*

Vasoactive intestinal peptide

Vasoactive intestinal peptide (**VIP**) is a digestive system peptide that is also located in some neurons that use acetylcholine (e.g. the parasympathetic nervous system stimulation of salivary glands), where it potentiates the action of acetylcholine. It would appear that VIP in the brain is likely to have a neuromodulatory role, not causing direct effects itself but modifying the effects of other neurotransmitters.

Substance P and substance K

Substance P and **substance K** are two peptides derived from the same pre-cursor molecule, the protein **protachykinin**.

Substance P was the first neuropeptide discovered. It is the neuro-transmitter of the grey matter at the back of the cord (called the dorsal horn). Here it functions on the main pain pathways from the periphery to the cord (i.e. the first sensory, or afferent, neuron). In the brain, substance P is mostly concentrated in the substantia nigra, where it activates dopaminergic neurons, and in the hypothalamus; it is also found in association with serotonin neurons originating in the raphe nucleus (see serotonin). Substance P binds to **NK receptors** (**NK = neurokinin**, the chemical category to which substance P belongs). Three such receptors are known, NK_1, NK_2 and NK_3, all of which are metabotropic. Substance P may have some influence on mood and thus on depression. Using drugs to block specific substance P receptors, particularly NK_1, could therefore become a useful line of treat-ment in mood disorders (NK_1 is found in brain areas involved in stress and emotions). Substance K, although isolated and chemically analysed and with at least one receptor found in the brain, is poorly understood in terms of brain activity. *See page 46*

Somatostatin

Somatostatin is a peptide found in various sites within the nervous system, such as the sympathetic nervous system (along with noradrenaline) and the thalamus (along with GABA). It is also present in the dorsal root ganglion of the first (peripheral) sensory neuron, the cerebral cortex and the limbic system, including the hippocampus (Figure 3.15). It is also a peptide of the digestive system, where it inhibits the release of several digestion-related hormones. In the brain, somatostatin has a sedatory effect and increases the action of sedatory drugs such as the barbiturates. It appears to reduce the rate of firing of neurons and suppresses motor activity. Several forms of the molecule are known to have activity in humans, notably somatostatin-14, somatostatin-25 and somatostatin-28, where the number represents the amino acid content of the molecule.

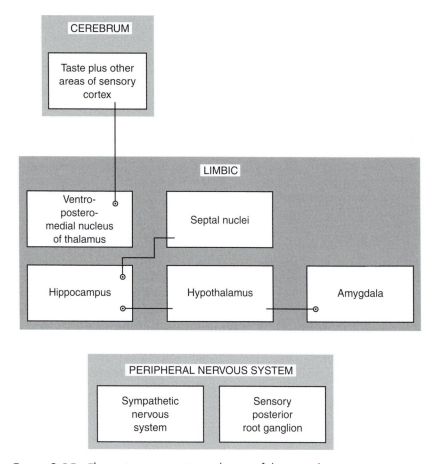

FIGURE 3.15 The main somatostatin pathways of the central nervous system.

Endogenous opioids

The chemistry of the brain involves the production of opiate-like sub-stances called **endogenous opioids**, proteins produced under pain or stress conditions which block pain at either **spinous** (spinal cord) or **supra-spinous** (brain stem) levels. Several classes of endogenous opioids are now known.

The **enkephalins** (Figure 3.16) are small peptides called **met-enkephalin** and **leu-enkephalin**, which are produced in response to minor pain, having an analgesic effects of about 2 minutes. **Beta-endorphin** (β-endorphin) is a larger peptide produced in response to more severe pain with an analgesia effect of around 4 hours or so.

The **dynorphins** (**dynorphin A**, **dynorphin B** and others) are intermediate peptides, and the **endomorphines** (**endomorphine-1** and **endomorphine-2**) are both small peptides. All of these naturally produced chemicals bind to opiate receptors in the upper cord and brain stem called **mu** (μ), **delta** (δ) and **kappa** (κ) receptors. Mu receptors may exist in two subtypes, μ_1 and μ_2, a distinction based on possible variations that may occur between the mu

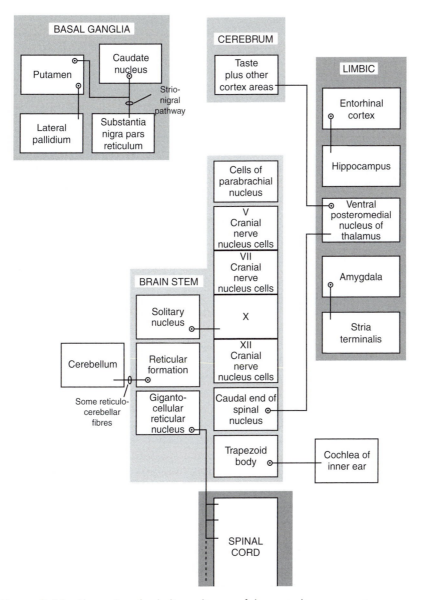

FIGURE 3.16 The main enkephalin pathways of the central nervous system.

receptors of the brain stem and the mu receptors of the respiratory centre. Delta receptors are similarly subdivided, with δ_1, δ_2, δ_{cx} and δ_{ncx} proposed. The δ_{cx} type is said to form a complex with mu receptors, whilst the δ_{ncx} does not form a complex with any other receptors.

Kappa receptor subtypes, κ_1 and κ_2, have become a complex issue, with other further subdivisions of each subtype proposed. Research will continue in this area, mainly because of the devastating problems caused by heroin and other opiate addictions and the need to find a solution to this problem. This work will eventually identify and classify many more subtypes of

TABLE 3.2 The affinity of endogenous opiates for opiate receptors

Endogenous opiate	High affinity	Low affinity	Negligible affinity
Enkephalin	δ	μ	κ
β- Endorphins	μ, δ, $κ_2$	Other κ	
Dynorphins	κ	μ, δ	
Endomorphine	μ		

the opiate receptors with a view to finding antagonist drugs that will prevent the opiates from binding. The affinity of the endogenous opiates for the various opiate receptors, where this has been established, is shown in Table 3.2.

Other neurotransmitters

Acetylcholine

Acetylcholine (ACh) is one of the earliest known synaptic ligands. Its production requires the enzyme **choline acetyltransferase (ChAT)**, which uses **choline** derived immediately from the extracellular fluid around the neuron and transfers an **acetyl group** to it to form ACh (Figure 3.17). Choline from dietary sources must be delivered to the brain by the blood, and therefore the supply of choline determines the amount of ACh that can be produced. Only **cholinergic** neurons (i.e. those that respond to ACh) contain ChAT and are therefore capable of producing ACh. These include **lower motor neurons (LMNs)** that use ACh at the **neuromuscular junction** (i.e. synapses between LMNs and muscle cells). ACh is produced in *See page 24* the neuronal cell body and moved to the synapse by axonal transport. After release into the synapse and binding to receptors, ACh is broken down while still within the cleft by another enzyme, **acetylcholinesterase (AChE)**. This releases the choline again from the molecule and much of this choline is returned to the presynaptic bulb and reused. The remaining **acetic acid** is excreted.

In the brain, acetylcholine is concentrated in the corpus striatum, with some found in the cerebrum, the nucleus accumbens, the limbic system

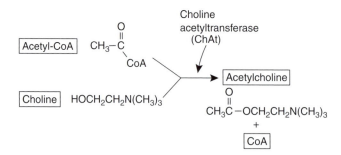

FIGURE 3.17 The synthesis of acetylcholine. The products are boxed with their chemical structure shown. The only enzyme (unboxed) labels the arrow.

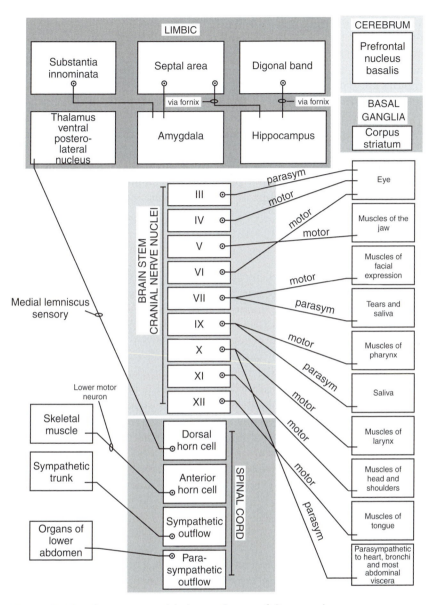

FIGURE 3.18 The main acetylcholine pathways of the central nervous system.

including the hippocampus, and parts of the brain stem, especially some of the cranial nerve nuclei (Figure 3.18).

Cholinergic receptors

Cholinergic receptors, i.e. those which bind acetylcholine, occur in two forms, **nicotinic** and **muscarinic**. Muscarine and nicotine are plant alkaloids which bind to the respective receptor. The nicotinic (N) receptor is ionotropic, causing the *direct* opening of membrane channels used by a range of cations, mostly Na^+ and Ca^{2+}. Nicotinic receptors are found mostly within the spinal cord, in the autonomic nervous system (ANS) and at the neuromuscular junction, but are less commonly found in the brain. Subtypes of nicotinic receptors are the N-m, found at the neuromuscular junction, and the N-n, found at the ganglion synapse of the ANS.

The muscarinic (M) receptors are metabotropic; they regulate potassium ion channels *indirectly* by first affecting the secondary messenger **cAMP**, and this in turn affects the ion channels. The subtypes of muscarinic receptors are M_1, M_2, M_3, M_4 and M_5. The functions of these subtypes vary, but they generally cause excitation in the postsynaptic membrane. They are more common than nicotinic receptors in the brain, occurring both as postsynaptic and autoreceptors.

Histamine

Histamine is known as a chemical agent outside the brain that induces inflammation when released from storage in mast cells or platelets. It is synthesised from the dietary amino acid **histidine** using the enzyme **histidine decarboxylase**, which requires **vitamin B_6 (pyroxidine)** to function. Histamine is also known as a neurotransmitter in the brain, but because it cannot cross the blood–brain barrier from the body to the brain, histamine must be synthesised within the brain. The hypothalamus has the greatest concentration of histidine decarboxylase found in the brain. Since the amino acid histidine can cross the blood–brain barrier, histamine can be produced in areas of the brain that have this enzyme, particularly the hypothalamus. Histamine is also found in a pathway extending from the brain stem to the cerebral cortex via the median forebrain bundle and in the hippocampus (Figure 3.19). Histamine is involved in the brain's control of alertness, part of the sleep–wake cycle, and in the mechanisms that regulate nausea and vomiting in the brain stem.

See page 114

Histamine receptors

Histamine receptors are of three known classes, H_1, H_2 and H_3; they are all metabotropic and are found in brain tissue. The H_1 receptor is found in both the brain stem and cerebral cortex, the two areas linked by the histaminergic median forebrain bundle mentioned above. Because of histamine's role in the control of alertness of the cerebrum, antihistamines (or H_1 antagonists), which are able to cross the blood–brain barrier, can cause drowsiness as a side-effect. H_2 receptors are found largely outside the brain on hydrochloric acid (HCl)-producing cells of the stomach wall, where the binding of histamine increases HCl production. In the brain, H_2 receptors are found in the same sites as H_1. H_3 receptors are found in the brain as a presynaptic autoreceptor on histaminergic neurons, allowing feedback to the presynaptic bulb on histamine release.

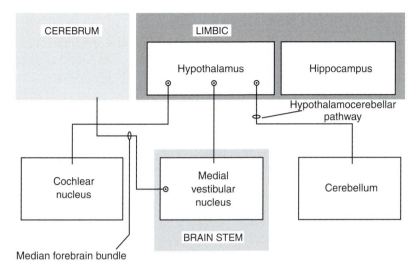

FIGURE 3.19 The main histamine pathways of the central nervous system.

Key points

Neurotransmitters and receptors

- Neurotransmitters are the chemical agents released from the presynaptic bulb into the synaptic cleft.
- Most neurotransmitters fall into three main groups: amines, amino acids and peptides.
- Activity at the synapse is due to the function of the receptor to which a neurotransmitter binds. The same neurotransmitter is often seen to produce different effects by binding to different receptors.
- Some receptors are postsynaptic, part of the *postsynaptic* membrane, others are autoreceptors on the *presynaptic* membranes or other parts of the neuron.
- Autoreceptors are thought to provide feedback information to the presynaptic bulb to regulate further neurotransmitter release.
- Some receptors are ionotropic; they control the opening or closing of a particular ion channel.
- Other receptors, called metobotrophic, cause changes in the metabolism of the postsynaptic cell.

Amine neurotransmitters

- Dopaminergic neurons and receptors are found in the basal ganglia (the nigrostriatal pathway) and the limbic system (mesolimbic pathway), and are involved in mental health symptoms and drug treatments.
- Serotonergic and adrenergic neurons and receptors are found in the diffuse modulatory pathways of the brain stem, and are involved in the cause and drug treatment of mood disorders.

Amino acid neurotransmitters

- Gamma-aminobutyric acid (GABA) is an important inhibitory neuro-transmitter, which is partly implicated in epilepsy. The $GABA_A$ receptor is a major site for the action of some drugs used in psychiatry.

References

Bear M. F., Connors B. W. and Paradiso M. A. (1996) *Neuroscience, Exploring the Brain*. Williams and Wilkins, Baltimore.

Blows W. T. (2000) Neurotransmitters of the brain: serotonin, noradrenaline (norepinephrine) and dopamine. *Journal of Neuroscience Nursing*, **32** (4): 234–238.

Carlson N. (2001) *Physiology of Behavior* (7th edn). Allyn and Bacon, Boston.

Nemeroff C. B. (1998) The neurobiology of depression. *Scientific American*: 28–35.

Wild G. C. and Benzel E. C. (1994) *Essentials of Neurochemistry*. Jones and Bartlett Publishers, Boston.

Chapter 4

Hormones and mental health

- Introduction: hormones, form and function
- The pituitary hormones
- The thyroid hormones
- Hormones from the adrenal cortex
- Hormones from the adrenal medulla
- The sex hormones
- Key points

Introduction: hormones, form and function

Hormones are chemical messengers: they move from one part of the body to another in the blood and have an effect, often stimulatory, on a *target* organ or tissue. The brain is the target organ for a range of hormones that have influence over neuronal growth and development as well as function.

Hormones are the products of **endocrine glands**, which are glands that secrete their products directly into the blood. Hormones are of two basic types, the protein hormones (the **peptides**) and the lipid (or fat-based) hormones (the **steroids**). In order to work, a hormone must first bind to a receptor site that is associated with the target cell. Cells without receptors for a specific hormone are not targets for that hormone. Peptide hormones are too large to penetrate the cell membrane and must therefore bind to receptors on the cell surface. Steroid hormones can pass through the membrane and bind with receptors within the cell cytoplasm or the nucleus (Figure 4.1). Receptors for hormones, like those for neurotransmitters, are usually proteins, coded by and synthesised from gene sequences within the

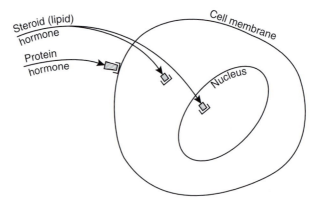

FIGURE 4.1 Hormones and receptors. Protein hormones are too large to enter the cell, so they bind to surface receptors. Steroid (lipid) hormones are smaller and so they can enter the cell and bind to receptors inside the cytoplasm or nucleus.

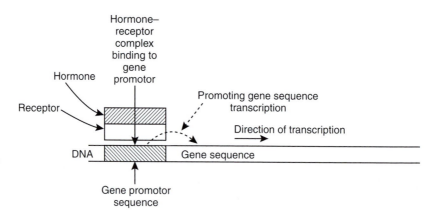

FIGURE 4.2 The complex of hormone and receptor affects gene transcription by interacting with the gene promotor sequence of the deoxyribonucleic acid (DNA).

target cell **DNA (deoxyribonucleic acid)**. DNA is the molecule housed inside the nucleus of most cells and forms the genes, the blueprints on which all cellular proteins and other characteristics are based. Cells therefore have the ability to increase (upregulate) or decrease (downregulate) their receptor numbers by activating or deactivating the appropriate genes. This affects the sensitivity of that cell to the effects of the hormone; since up-regulation can bind more hormone, down-regulation binds less hormone.

On binding to the receptor, the hormone–receptor complex effects changes within the cell usually by binding to a **gene promoter** sequence on the DNA and initiating transcription of the gene (Figure 4.2). **Gene transcription** involves the assembly of an **RNA (ribonucleic acid)** molecule, the first step in protein synthesis. In this way hormones arriving at the cell trigger a wave of protein synthesis which will alter in some way the activity of that cell. In neurons this change in activity is likely to influence the response of the cell to action potentials or to neurotransmitters.

As the functional component of the endocrine system, hormones are regulated by **feedback mechanisms** that influence their production and release from the gland. Feedback mechanisms are a part of general **homeostasis** by which the body maintains a stable internal environment that promotes optimum function of its organs. Homeostasis is critical in many areas such as temperature control, electrolyte, fluid and acid–base balance. Many nursing observations are carried out in order to monitor the function and effectiveness of specific homeostatic mechanisms; observations such as recording of the pulse rate, blood pressure and temperature (Blows 2001). Homeostasis operates through the two major communication systems of the body, the endocrine and nervous systems. Close collaboration between these two systems is responsible for regulating most of the functions of the cells and tissues through a wide variety of situations, a collaboration known as the **neuroendocrine response**. Disturbance of homeostasis causes biochemical and other imbalances which seriously upset the normal functioning of various organs, not least the brain. Some disorders of homeostasis involving hormones can cause mental symptoms for which the hormonal levels of the blood require investigation.

The pituitary hormones

The pituitary hormones were listed in Chapter 1 because they are subject to hypothalamic control. As will be seen in the following pages, some disorders of the pituitary gland can disrupt the function of other endocrine glands and the resulting change in hormonal levels can cause mental symptoms. Important examples of this are changes in **thyroid-stimulating hormone (TSH)**, which controls levels of thyroid hormone in the blood, and in **adrenocorticotropic hormone (ACTH)**, which influences adrenal cortex function by stimulating cortisol production (Figure 4.3).

The thyroid hormones

The thyroid hormones occur in two forms, **triiodothyronine (T3)** and **tetraiodothyronine (T4)** (Figure 4.3). **Iodine** is a major component of this hormone and the two forms have respectively three and four atoms of iodine per molecule. They are a product of the thyroid gland, which is situated in the neck, on top of the trachea and below the larynx. Thyroid hormones are essential for the growth, development and metabolic function of many tissues, not least the brain. In normal tissues, these hormones maintain normal metabolism within the cell. Changes in mental function appear if the levels of thyroid hormone are too low or too high. Disorders of thyroid level may be *primary* (i.e. affecting the gland itself), or *secondary* (i.e. caused by abnormal changes in TSH level from the anterior pituitary gland).

Hypothyroidism, in which the blood level of thyroid hormone is too low, is sometimes called **myxoedema**. It is most common in females over the age of 40 years. Failure to produce enough of this hormone can result in a number of symptoms which could be misinterpreted as a true mental disorder. Patients with myxoedema suffer lethargy, depression, personality

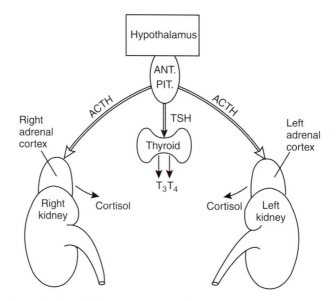

Figure 4.3 The hypothalamo–pituitary–adrenal (HPA) axis, where adrenocorticotropic hormone (ACTH) from the anterior pituitary stimulates cortisol production. The hypothalamo–pituitary–thyroid (HPT) axis, where thyroid-stimulating hormone (TSH) stimulates the release of the thyroid hormones T_3 and T_4.

changes and psychotic episodes known as *myxoedema madness*. This is manifested as paranoia, hallucinations and delirium.

Hypothyroid disorders are occasionally associated with depressive mood disorders and about 10% of depressed patients with lethargy are also hypothyroid. Thyroid hormone treatment is sometimes used in addition to antidepressant drugs to improve the patient's response to the antidepressant therapy. Such a combination is sometimes used in those patients who quickly rotate between the depressed and manic phases of bipolar depression. The antimanic drug *lithium* can predispose to hypothyroid states and therefore monitoring of thyroid function during lithium treatment is important to avoid complications. Neonatal hypothyroidism puts the newly born infant at risk of developmental brain function failure, known as **cretinism**, a serious problem that can be corrected if recognised from birth and treated with thyroid hormone.

Hyperthyroidism, or **thyrotoxicosis**, is the production of excess thyroid hormone by the thyroid gland. Thyrotoxicosis refers to a cluster of related disorders all of which ultimately release excess hormone into the blood. These disorders are either primary, caused by a problem with the thyroid itself, or secondary, resulting from a response by a normal thyroid to too much TSH from the pituitary gland. In either case the patient shows anxiety, agitation and delirium, with nervous excitability, irritability, insomnia and other psychotic manifestations. If the hormone excess is severe, memory loss and disorientation can occur, with manic excitability, delusions and hallucinations. Stress seems to be a causative factor, theoretically owing to excessive use of the endocrine system during childhood trauma (e.g. loss of

See page 181
See page 198

See page 142

parents, economic hardship, rivalry with siblings) (Kaplan and Sudock 1996). It becomes important, therefore, for all patients suffering from 'anxiety' to have their blood thyroid hormone and TSH levels measured to exclude a thyroid problem.

Hormones from the adrenal cortex

The adrenal glands, situated on top of the kidneys, have an *outer* **cortex** and an *inner* **medulla**. The cortex produces several steroidal hormones based on cholesterol derived from the blood (Figure 4.4). There are several hormonal groups produced by the cortex, including the **mineralocorticoids** (those hormones active on minerals); the **glucocorticoids** (those hormones influencing blood glucose levels); and the sex hormones for males (**androgens**) and females (**estrogens**) (Figure 4.4).

Cortisol is a glucocorticoid, the production of which is stimulated by ACTH from the anterior pituitary gland. Cortisol has several functions, notably raising the blood glucose level by its anti-insulin effects, and it helps to protect cells against the adverse effects of stress.

Excess cortisol occurs in the disorder **Cushing syndrome** and after prolonged corticosteroid drug treatment. The disorder occurs more often in women than in men and causes a similar state to that of bipolar depression (Rosenzweig *et al.* 1999), with insomnia, loss of emotions and energy, and attempted suicide in about 10% of untreated patients. Alternatively, the patient's mood may swing into euphoria, agitation, mania and delirium, with psychotic symptoms such as hallucinations. Depression may also follow withdrawal from long-term steroid therapy, this being one reason for a long period of gradual rather than sudden reduction of dosage from these drugs.

See page 181

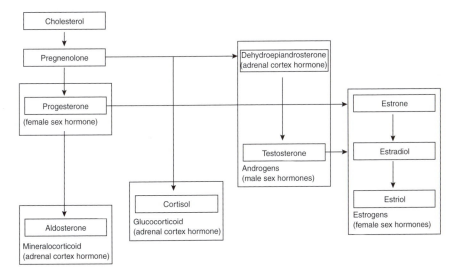

FIGURE 4.4 Flow diagram of the production of various steroidal (lipid-based) hormones from cholesterol in the adrenal cortex, including cortisol, aldosterone, the female oestrogens and the male androgens.

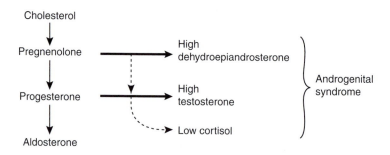

FIGURE 4.5 Adrenogenital syndrome, caused by excessive androgens (testosterone and dehydroepiandrosterone) in conjunction with low cortisol.

Some women with Cushing syndrome may show a degree of **masculinisation**, growing unwanted hair and losing their menstrual periods (**amenorrhoea**), and this can add to their depression. Men with this condition can become impotent and lose their hair.

Addison disease is an insufficiency in cortisol production from the adrenal cortex. Lack of cortisol results in the patient becoming tired, lethargic and depressed and sometimes showing psychotic symptoms. The person may also develop delirium and confusion. Generally the mental symptoms are milder that those seen in Cushing syndrome. The problem may not reside in the adrenal gland itself but could be a failure of adrenocorticotropic *See page 66* hormone (ACTH) from the pituitary gland. Treatment with corticosteroid supplements is essential for life.

Production of cortisol is also severely reduced in a condition called **adrenogenital syndrome** (Figure 4.5). The poor secretion of cortisol can be caused by low activity of either of the enzymes **21-hydroxylase** or **11β-hydroxylase**, both of which are essential for the pathway that leads to cortisol (Figure 4.4). This is a **congenital** defect; that is, the person is born with the enzyme error, the consequences of which are a corresponding increase in the synthesis of androgens. In the female fetus this causes Addison disease, the excess androgens having a masculinising effect at the same time. The 'girl', while being genetically female, develops male-like external genitalia, making gender difficult to determine (**pseudohermaphroditism**). The excess testosterone produced may also have a masculinising effect on the girl's *See page 71* brain, causing a mental conflict of identity or 'self'. In a male fetus with this condition, the Addison disease is accompanied by advanced sexual development in early puberty.

A similar condition, **adrenogenitalism** (Figure 4.6), occurs in the fetus when the pituitary gland produces too much ACTH. The excessive stimulation of the adrenal cortex results in higher than normal production of testosterone, the main male androgen. Cortisol production in this situation remains normal since all the enzymes involved in the steroid hormone pathways are functioning. The stimulation of the cortex causes **hyperplasia** (excessive cellular growth) within the cortex of the gland. This is an **autosomal** *See page 74* **recessive** disorder, again causing masculinisation of the female fetus (pseudohermaphroditism) with male-like external genitalia. The male fetus

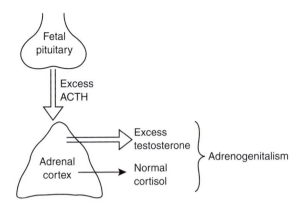

FIGURE 4.6 Adrenogenitalism, caused by excessive ACTH driving testosterone production to excess, while cortisol remains normal.

with this condition has excessive sexual development, except for smaller-than-average testes, which remain underdeveloped owing to the negative feedback from the high adrenal testosterone. Testosterone stimulates growth, so androgenital children of both sexes are generally taller than their peers, but as bone growth is stopped prematurely they are therefore shorter than average as adults. The mental effect is again one of conflict concerning sexual identity and this may need to be addressed by both physical and psychological treatment.

Hormones from the adrenal medulla

The hormones produced by the adrenal medulla are the **catecholamines**, adrenaline and noradrenaline. Adrenaline has sympathomimetic activity, that is, it increases the functions of the sympathetic nervous system (Figure 4.7). The physical symptoms of excessive stimulation of the sympathetic nervous system include an increase in the heart rate, sweating, tremor and insomnia. The mental symptoms include apprehension or even fear leading to panic, all of which give a clinical picture of anxiety attacks. Differentiation between excessive catecholamine production and true anxiety may be achieved by measuring the blood adrenaline levels, although anxiety itself may cause increased release of this hormone. A rare cause of high levels of adrenaline in the blood is an adrenaline-producing tumour of the medulla called a **phaeochromocytoma**.

See page 43

See page 18

See page 146

The sex hormones

The **estrogens** and **androgens** are the sex hormone groups for females and males respectively. There are three estrogen hormones and two androgen hormones. The female estrogens are **estradiol, estrone and estriol** and the male androgens are **testosterone** and **dehydroepiandrosterone** (Figure 4.4). Estradiol is the most potent of the estrogens, while testosterone is the most potent of the androgens. They are all synthesised from **cholesterol** via

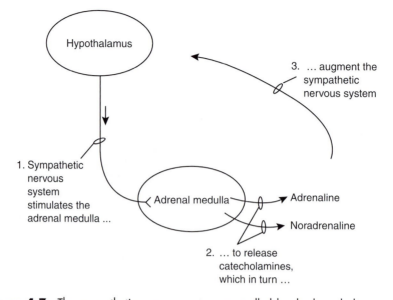

FIGURE 4.7 The sympathetic nervous system, controlled by the hypothalamus, can increase the production of catecholamines (adrenaline and noradrenaline) from the adrenal medulla. These, in turn, augment the sympathetic nervous system.

a pathway which includes the production of the other steroidal hormones, **cortisol**, **progesterone** and **aldosterone** (Figure 4.4). Following puberty, the female ovary produces most of the estrogen, while the male testes produces most of the testosterone. However, in addition, trace quantities of both the estrogens and the androgens are produced and released from the **adrenal cortex** in both sexes. Females produce small quantities of androgens and males produce small quantities of estrogens. This is a vestige of the past life of the growing fetus, when the adrenal cortex was the sole producer of these substances. Both these hormonal groups have a multitude of target tissues and organs around the body, including the brain, where they have a profound influence on functional and sexual organisation. Estrogen creates a 'feminine' brain, while testosterone forms a 'masculine' brain. It is important to note that these hormonal organisational effects happen at very precise and critical moments in fetal brain development. After this critical point the hormonal influence over the brain is of a different nature; that of influencing behavioural patterns, in particular sexual behaviour, and mood. High levels of testosterone are known to influence aggression in males, while estrogen reduces aggression. Low levels of testosterone appear to result from stress and are linked to nervousness, bad temper and depressed moods in men (the so-called **irritable male syndrome**) (Nowak 2002). Postmenopausal loss of estrogen in women can lead to anxiety, loss of confidence, forgetfulness and even depression.

The hypothalamus is involved is sexual behaviour and perinatal exposure to androgens in the male causes a larger preoptic region of the hypothalamus than in females (Kimura 1992). In fact, the anterior hypothalamus shows

See page 71

See page 148

TABLE 4.1 Sex differences in the brain in terms of task performance

MALE orientated brain (skills at which males are better than females)	FEMALE orientated brain (skills at which females are better than males)
• Spatial tasks, especially rotational skills • Mathematical reasoning • Navigational skills (e.g. map reading) • Target-directed skills, such as guiding or intercepting projectiles (e.g. dart throwing)	• Perceptual speed, i.e. rapid identification of matching items • Arithmetical calculations • Precision manual skills (e.g. embroidery) • Verbal fluency • Recall of landmarks along a route

significant **sexual dimorphism** (i.e. variation between the sexes) in the *pattern of synaptic connections* found there. This part of the brain has been called the **sexually dimorphic nucleus**. This structural variation is achieved through exposure to sex hormones before, during and after birth. It is also important to note that at such an early stage of development the source of the estrogen or testosterone cannot be the ovaries or testes, as they only begin production much later in life. Early production of the sex hormones relies on the adrenal cortex, which begins releasing significant levels in early life but reduces production later.

The differences between the two brains are demonstrable in various tests that male and female subjects are asked to perform. However, it is not possible to say exactly how each hormone effects changes in neural tissues. The results of the tests show a trend in the types of skills each sex is better equipped to do (Table 4.1). While male brains are physically larger than female brains, women have a greater concentration of grey matter cells (or neurons) in the areas concerned with communication. These areas are the dorsolateral prefrontal cortex (involved in memory and initiative: 23% more cells) and the superior temporal gyrus (involved in listening: 13% more cells).

The sexual orientation of the brain is dependent on two factors, genetic heredity patterns and prenatal exposure to hormones (androgens in males and estrogens in females) (Carlson 2001). Male brains show a greater degree of lateralisation than those of females, designating one hemisphere for a task rather than both. This can be a handicap in circumstances where the designated hemisphere becomes damaged. In males the task is often lost altogether, while females can switch to the other hemisphere. A typical example is damage to the speech centre in the left hemisphere, where **aphasia** (loss of speech) occurs four times more often in males (who cannot switch to the right side) than in females (who can often make the switch). Lateralisation does not necessarily make the performance of a skill any better. In female brains there is increased overlap between the hemisphere functions for the verbal skills and women do better in these skills than men. There are also other physical differences in the brain between the sexes, the significance of which is not always understood:

- Females have longer temporal lobes than males.
- The female posterior corpus callosum (connecting the left hemisphere with the right hemisphere) is bulbous and wide compared to that in the male, which is cylindrical and uniform in width throughout its length.
- The female brain is more tightly packed with grey matter.

Key points

Hormones

- Hormones are chemical messengers; they have an effect on a *target* organ or tissue.
- The brain is the target organ for many hormones, influencing neuronal growth, development and function.
- Hormones come from endocrine glands, and are of two basic types, proteins and lipids (called steroids).
- A hormone must bind to a receptor site on the target cell.
- The hormone–receptor complex changes the cell by binding to DNA, and causing transcription of a gene.

Thyroid hormones

- Thyroid hormone occurs in two forms, triiodothyronine (T_3) and tetraiodothyronine (T_4). Iodine is a major component of this hormone.
- Hypothyroidism (or myxoedema) is too low a blood level of thyroid hormone, which causes depression, lethargy, personality changes and psychotic episodes (myxoedema madness).
- Lithium can cause hypothyroidism, and patients should be monitored for thyroid function.
- Neonatal hypothyroidism, leading to brain developmental failure, is known at cretinism. It is corrected by treatment with thyroid hormone.
- Hyperthyroidism (thyrotoxicosis) is excess thyroid hormone in the blood causing memory loss, disorientation, manic excitability, delusions and hallucinations.

Adrenal cortex hormones

- Cortisol is a glucocorticoid from the adrenal cortex. Production is stimulated by adrenocorticotropic hormone (ACTH) from the anterior pituitary gland.
- Excess cortisol causes Cushing's syndrome causing depression-like symptoms, insomnia, energy loss and emotional flattening. Sufferers may have mood swings with euphoria, and delirium with hallucinations.
- Addison disease is a lack of cortisol, causing tiredness, lethargy and depression, and sometimes delirium and confusion.
- Adrenogenital syndrome is a lack of cortisol due to low activity of either of the enzymes of the pathway leading to cortisol production. This is a congenital defect. The synthesis of androgens increases, causing a

masculinising effect in the female fetus (pseudohermaphroditism) and a mental conflict of gender identity. The male fetus shows signs of advanced sexual development at a young age.

- Adrenogenitalism occurs when a fetus produces too much ACTH from the pituitary gland, resulting in raised levels of testosterone. Hyperplasia is an autosomal recessive disorder that causes masculinisation of the female fetus and excessive sexual development of the male fetus.
- The female estrogens are estradiol, estrone and estriol, and the male androgens are testosterone and dehydroepiandrosterone. Estradiol is the most potent of the estrogens, whilst testosterone is the most potent of the androgens.
- Estrogen creates a 'feminine' brain, whilst testosterone forms a 'masculine' brain.

References

Blows W. T. (2001) *The Biological Basis of Nursing: Clinical Observations*. Routledge, London.

Carlson N. R. (2001) *Physiology of Behavior* (7th edn), Allyn and Bacon, Boston.

Kaplan H. I. and Sudock B. J. (1996) *Concise Textbook of Clinical Psychiatry*. Williams and Wilkins, Baltimore.

Kimura D. (1992) Sex Differences in the Brain. http://www.scientificamerican.com/2002/0602mind/0602kimura.html

Nowak R. (2002) Men behaving sadly. *New Scientist*, 173 (2332) (2 March 2002): 4.

Rosenzweig M. R., Leiman A. L. and Breedlove S. M. (1999) *Biological Psychology, an Introduction to Behavioural, Cognitive, and Clinical Neuroscience* (2nd edn). Sinauer Associates, Sunderland, MA.

Chapter 5

Genetic disorders affecting mental health

- Introduction
- Chromosomes and genes
- Disorders of inheritance
- Chromosomal disorders
- Genetic disorders
- Sex chromosomes
- Key points

Introduction

A better understanding of the genetic component of many diseases is nowadays crucial to unravelling the pathology of the disease and improving its management. This is particularly true in the case of mental health disorders. As key persons in the management of these disorders, nurses will need a good working knowledge of the subject if they are to participate in counselling, drug treatment and research intended to improve treatment and care. This chapter therefore provides a brief introduction to human genetics and an overview of the genetic aspects of disorders that nurses will commonly encounter.

Chromosomes and genes

The human **karyotype**, or chromosome 'set', is made up of 46 chromosomes arranged as shown in Figure 5.1. Forty-four of these chromosomes pair up to make 22 pairs of **autosomes**, which regulate many different body

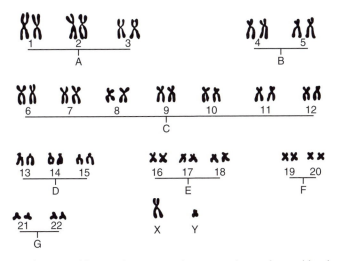

FIGURE 5.1   The normal human karyotype (this is a male, as denoted by the Y chromosome). A normal karyotype has 46 chromosomes, 22 pairs of autosomes (1 to 22) and one pair of sex chromosomes.

activities. The chromosomes making up the final pair are the sex chromosomes – X and Y in males, X and X in females. The chromosomes carry our **genes**, some of the largest carrying more than 4500!

Of each pair of chromosomes, one is inherited from the mother, the other from the father. Each pair of autosomes therefore consists of two chromosomes that are structurally the same, carrying an identical arrangement of corresponding genes. For this reason they are known as **homologous autosomes** (homologous = similar, corresponding to). The genes that occur on one chromosome of a pair also occur in the same positions on the other chromosome of the same pair. Alternative versions of the same gene are called **alleles**, one allele on each chromosome. Although they are the same gene, because they come from different parents they are likely to carry different **traits**. The difference between *genes* and *traits* is highlighted by the following example: the gene for eye colour carries different traits according to which parent it comes from. In the case of eye colour, one gene could carry the trait for blue eyes, the other gene the trait for green eyes. So, eye colour is the gene, while blue or green are the traits. If two different eye colour traits are present in the same karyotype, which one will become the true colour of the eye in that individual? In other words, which gene will be expressed into the **phenotype** (the physical body)? The answer to the question depends on which gene is **dominant** and which is **recessive**. Dominant genes are always expressed into the phenotype when present at either one or both alleles (Figure 5.2). Their traits therefore become a physical feature of the person. When the same genes (and the same traits) are present at both alleles they are described as **homozygous**. When different genes (and therefore different traits) are present at the alleles they are known as **heterozygous**. Recessive genes are only expressed into the phenotype when they are present at both alleles, i.e. when no dominant gene is present (Figure 5.3). A

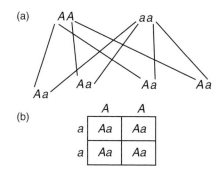

FIGURE 5.2 Dominant gene inheritance. Capital letter equals dominant gene, small letter equals recessive gene. Homozygous parents (*AA*, i.e. both dominant genes; or *aa*, both recessive genes) will have offspring that are all mixed (*Aa*, i.e. mixed dominant and recessive). Shown as a cross-over and as a punnett square.

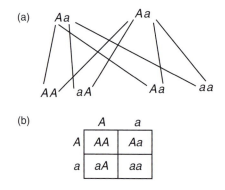

FIGURE 5.3 Recessive gene inheritance. Capital letter equals dominant gene, small letter equals recessive gene. Heterozygous parents (*Aa*, i.e. mixed dominant and recessive genes) have 25% chance of having an *AA* offspring (i.e. pure dominant genes), 50% chance of having an *Aa* offspring (i.e. mixed genes), and 25% chance of having an *aa* offspring (purely recessive). This last child shows recessive traits (or a recessive genetic disorder) that has missed one or more generations. Shown as a cross-over and as a punnett square.

recessive gene at only one allele will not be expressed and the alternative dominant gene will determine the physical trait. Two different dominant traits, one at each allele, may both be expressed into the phenotype as **co-dominant** genes, resulting in some kind of mixture of both traits in the phenotype of the individual.

Genes demonstrate varying degrees of **penetrance** – that is, the amount to which each individual gene contributes to the completed body (the phenotype). Genes showing complete penetrance achieve maximum influence over the phenotype. Incomplete penetrance occurs where the gene is only minimally activated, resulting in a weak influence on the phenotype. Dominant genes will often show a high degree of penetrance whenever they are present, but recessive genes will have little or no penetrance unless they exist at both alleles (i.e. no dominant gene is present). The amount of penetrance that a *mutated* (or abnormal) gene demonstrates is an indication of its influence on the severity and course of several important mental health disorders. However, those genes of low-level penetrance may still be passed on to future generations of the same family where the gene's penetrance may be altered and increased.

Genes are stretches of **deoxyribonucleic acid (DNA)** found within the **chromatin** that makes up the chromosomes, and this DNA provides a code for producing specific proteins. Through the DNA, genes determine three important things about proteins:

- the proteins that will be produced;
- the amino acids that will be present in the final protein;
- the sequence of amino acids in the protein.

DNA comprises four chemical **bases: adenine (A), thymine (T), guanine (G)** and **cytosine (C)**, usually represented by their first letter as shown in brackets here. These bases form groups of three along the DNA called **codons,** and each codon codes for one specific amino acid in the final protein; for example, the codon GCA (guanine, cytosine and adenine) codes for the amino acid **alanine** (Figure 5.4). The types, numbers and sequence of the codons determines the type, numbers and sequence of the amino acids in the completed protein.

Genes have a particular site where they are found on the chromosome, called the gene **locus** (or **gene slot**). This locus is specified by giving the chromosome number first, followed by the arm of the chromosome (p = short arm; q = long arm), and then the site number along that arm where the

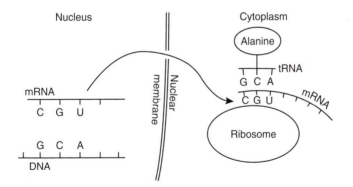

Figure 5.4 The genetic code for alanine. GCA (guanine–cytosine–adenine) on the DNA codes for the amino acid alanine by first forming the opposite code on messenger RNA (mRNA). The opposite of G is C, but the opposite of A is U (uracil) in RNA. U replaces the T (thymine) used in DNA. The mRNA leaves the nucleus and binds with a ribosome. Transfer RNAs (tRNAs) bear the same codes of bases as the original DNA codons (triplets of bases) in the DNA in the nucleus; of the case shown here it is GCA, coding for alanine. Repeating this along the DNA molecule, with different codes for different amino acids, forms a string of amino acids at the ribosome called a protein.

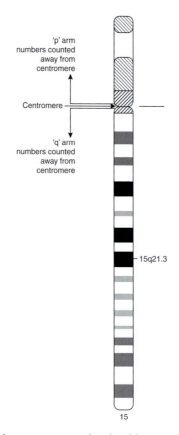

'p' arm
numbers counted
away from
centromere

Centromere

'q' arm
numbers counted
away from
centromere

15q21.3

15

FIGURE 5.5 The gene locus. Genes are localised by a code using first the chromo-some number (here it is chromosome 15), then the arm, represented by 'p' for the short arm, 'q' for the long arm, and then the number counted away from the centromere. So 15q21.3 identifies the long arm of the 15th chromosome at point 21.3 from the centromere.

gene is located (see Figure 5.5). As an example, take the gene locus 15q21.3, which means it is on the 15th chromosome, in the long arm (q) at the site numbered 21.3 counted away from the chromosome's **centromere**, i.e. the point where the two chromatin strands join. The higher the number, the farther from the centromere the gene is sited (see Figure 5.5).

The proteins derived from the genetic code are of various types. They could be, for example:

- structural proteins involved in building the cells of the body;
- enzymes involved in the metabolism of cells;
- hormones involved in the regulation of body functions;
- antibodies involved in the defence systems of the body.

This list alone illustrates the vital importance of genes in the construction, function and defence of the body and why gene errors can be so devastating to the individual. Most gene errors are **mutations**, where changes occur in the bases of the DNA resulting in a false code and therefore an error in the protein produced from that code. This faulty protein will no longer function properly. Mutations occur as a result of damage to DNA, caused either by chemicals or by radiation, that is beyond the capabilities of the DNA repair enzymes. These excellent enzyme systems (which we share in common with the elephant!) can repair most of the mutations that occur, but sometimes the damage is missed or is beyond repair. Mutations that are inherited from generation to generation are rarely repaired and may often go on to cause diseases. Mutations include the following DNA errors (Figure 5.6):

1 **Point mutations**, where a single base is swapped for another, in-correct, base. This has the effect of coding for the wrong amino acid in the protein, which therefore suffers a loss of function to varying degrees.

2 **Translocations**, where some DNA of one chromosome has switched position with another stretch of DNA from a second chromosome. As an example, a 9:21 translocation means that chromosomes 9 and 21 have switched parts of their DNA with each other. The DNA is now in the wrong place and activation of these codes is likely to cause either a faulty protein or no protein product at all.

3 **Deletions**, where some DNA is lost and chromosomes are there-fore incomplete. The loss of some, perhaps many, genes will be detri-mental to the function of the body, since some vital proteins cannot be produced.

4 **Duplication**, where a sequence of DNA is copied (as part of a chromo-some) and added onto the previously existing arm of a chromosome (Figure 5.6g).

5 **Inversion**, where DNA is turned upside down in the chromosome and may be coded backwards, causing disruption of both the code and the protein that results.

6 **Frame shifts**, where the codon is read incorrectly one base to the left or right of the correct reading frame. As an example, if the DNA sequence was . . . AACGCATT . . . , the normal codon reading might be AAC, then GCA, and so on. However, a frame shift might read ACG, CAT, . . . , i.e. it would be read one base along to the right. It could also be read one base along to the left, i.e. CGC, ATT and so on. The result of either shift is the incorrect reading of the codes, leading to the wrong amino acids being selected and the protein being wrongly constructed.

7 **Base sequence repeats** (the so-called **stuttering gene**), where one codon is repeated many times – often hundreds of times – resulting in a long chain of one type of amino acid on the end of the protein. This is seen in several mental health and neurological conditions, notably Huntington disease and possibly schizophrenia. The mechanism of how this error causes neurological and mental health problems is not fully determined. Not only do base sequence repeats occur as familial disorders (passed on through multiple generations of the same family), they also show the

THE BIOLOGICAL BASIS OF NURSING: MENTAL HEALTH

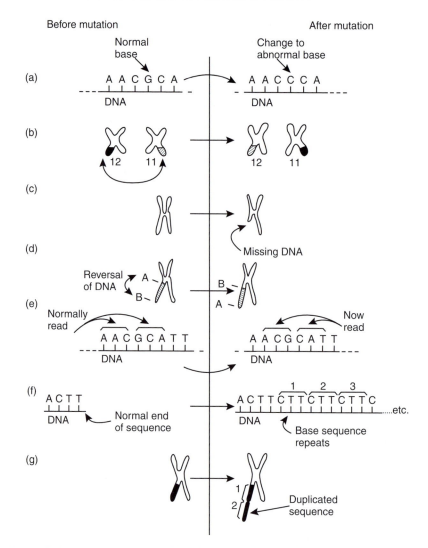

FIGURE 5.6 Genetic mutations. The left column shows before the mutation, the right column is after the mutation. (a) In a point mutation one base on the DNA is changed to a different one, creating a different code which introduces a different amino acid into the protein. (b) Translocation, in which a DNA sequence is swapped over between two chromosomes (shown here as an 11:12 translocation). (c). Deletion, in which a DNA sequence is lost entirely. (d). Inversion, in which a DNA sequence is reversed on the same chromosome (and thus will be read backwards). (e) Frame shift, where the normal DNA reading is moved one or more bases along (shown here as a single base shift normally read AAC, but now read ACG). This changes the amino acids in the protein. (f) Repeated base sequence, where the same base code is repeated many times (here it is CTT), resulting in a long tail of one kind of amino acid on the protein. (g) Duplication, where a DNA sequence is copied and attached to the end of a chromosome.

80

phenomenon of **anticipation**. In this the disorder comes on earlier, and shows increasingly severe symptoms, in each successive generation of individuals in that family, as each successive generation adds further to the repeats (see Huntington disease).

8 **Unstable sequence**, where a very large repeated base sequence, similar to but much longer than that found in (7) above, causes a complete loss of gene function. Fragile X syndrome is such a condition, resulting in some degree of mental retardation.

Disorders of inheritance

Autosomal gene mutations are responsible for a number of genetically inherited disorders and genetically **acquired** disorders (i.e. those where an individual has developed a gene error due to the damage and mutation of a previously normal gene). However, environmental factors are also likely to play an important role in some mental health disorders and these disorders are therefore usually classified as **polygenic**, where several genes are seen as interacting with one or several environmental factors to cause the disorder. In this sense, genes play a role that *increases the susceptibility* of an individual to develop a particular disorder, rather than causing the disorder directly. Whether the person develops the disorder or not may depend the environmental factors they encounter.

Inherited genetic disorders are said to be **familial**; that is, they are found in successive generations of the same family. In the case of *inherited* disorders, the gene error is passed on from parents to offspring through the sperm or ovum. In studies involving families affected by an inherited gene disorder the researcher will look at percentage risks between **first-degree relatives** (parents, brothers, sisters, sons or daughters) of an affected person. Studies of **second-degree relatives** (grandparents, aunts or uncles), or even **third-degree relatives** (e.g. cousins) of an affected person may also be of value in understanding the nature of the gene and its inheritance pattern. Studies of twins are particularly important when studying genetic inheritance, especially of **monozygotic (identical) twins** who have all their genes in common. Table 5.1 shows the approximate proportions of genes shared between an affected person and their various relatives. From this it can be seen that **nonidentical (dizygotic) twins** share the same amount of genes as ordinary brothers or sisters.

TABLE 5.1 Proportions of genes in common between relatives of different degrees

Relationship to affected person	Approximate percentage of shared genes
Monozygotic (MZ or identical) twin	100
Dizygotic (DZ or nonidentical) twin	50
First-degree relative (sibling, parent, son, daughter)	50
Second-degree relative (grandparent, aunt, uncle)	25
Third-degree relative (e.g. cousin)	12.5

For a discussion on the genes related to a specific mental disorder, see the chapter on that disorder; for example, the genes involved in depression are discussed in Chapter 9, those for schizophrenia in Chapter 8, and those for dementia in Chapter 12. Genes involved in Huntington and Parkinson's diseases are discussed in Chapter 11.

The most important difference between a genetic disorder and a chromosomal disorder is the number of genes involved. In genetic disorders there may be one or just a few genes at the root cause of a particular disease, whilst chromosomal disorders involve abnormalities of a whole or part of a chromosome, adding up to perhaps several thousand genes.

Chromosomal disorders

Two major chromosomal errors can result in mental health disorders: those that involve whole chromosomes and thus affect the number of chromosomes in the karyotype (e.g. trisomies and monosomies), and those that affect part of individual chromosomes without influencing the karyotype number (e.g. deletions).

Disorders of abnormal karyotype count

Several chromosomal abnormalities can occur that result in an abnormal karyotype chromosome count, where the normal value is 46 chromosomes. A **trisomy** is the occurrence of one extra chromosome attached to a pair, giving a karyotype of 47 chromosomes (Figure 5.7b). A **monosomy** is the occurrence of only one chromosome instead of a pair, giving a karyotype of 45 chromosomes (Figure 5.7a). Some trisomies and many monosomies do not survive; the individuals bearing them are subject to spontaneous abortion caused by nature. This is because either too much genetic material is

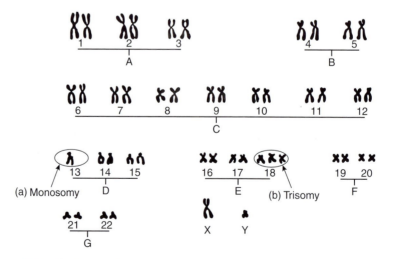

FIGURE 5.7 The human karyotype showing monosomy (here seen at chromosome 13) and trisomy (here seen at chromosome 18).

present (trisomies) or not enough is present (monosomies) to be compatible with life. The trisomies that *survive* to birth are those of autosomes 8, 9, 13, 18, 20, 21 and 22, while the only autosomal monosomy that survives is monosomy 21. Most of these phenotype abnormalities are associated with some degree of mental retardation and therefore may be seen by the psychiatric nurse at some time. Patients bearing several of them may survive to full term but are likely to die very young, sometimes within months of delivery.

Trisomy 8 (three number 8 chromosomes) results in an individual who is taller than average with a large skull and some mental retardation.

Trisomy 13 (three number 13 chromosomes) is called **Patau syndrome**. This occurs about once in every 5000 live births and causes severe physical abnormalities with profound mental retardation. Half of those born with this syndrome die within one month of their birth.

Trisomy 18 (three number 18 chromosomes) is called **Edward syndrome**. This is slightly more common than Patau syndrome, being present in one in 3000 live births. It causes various physical abnormalities, failure of growth and mental retardation. About 30% of cases will die before their first birthday.

A constant physical abnormality in these trisomy disorders is craniofacial malformation, such as cleft lip and palate, or more rarely **cyclopia** (the child is born with a single eye in the forehead, and this is often associated with an absent forebrain). New work is revealing a chemical link between the development of the brain and facial construction (Cohen 2000). Both the face and the brain are influenced in their formation by chemicals such as vitamin A, an influence which is somehow genetically controlled.

Down syndrome: trisomy 21

Trisomy 21 (three number 21 chromosomes instead of two) produces **Down syndrome** (Figure 5.8). This is more common than other trisomies, occurring on average in about one in 600 live births. The incidence of a Down syndrome child being born increases with maternal age: the older the mother is at the time of pregnancy the greater is the risk of Down syndrome. A typical risk pattern is seen in Table 5.2.

The extra chromosome is caused mostly by a **non-dysjunction**, where ovarian cell division results in abnormal separation of the chromosomes and one ovum retains both of the chromosomes 21. The older the woman becomes, the greater becomes the risk of non-dysjunction. The addition of a third chromosome 21 from the sperm on fertilisation results in the trisomy. Incidentally, should the normal sperm fertilise the other half of that ovum division – the half with no chromosome 21 – it would generate a monosomy 21 (having only the paternal chromosome 21).

Down syndrome results in a wide range of physical abnormalities and varying degrees of mental retardation. The physical abnormalities include a round skull on a short, broad neck, a flattened face and a prominent epicanthus of the eye (the upper lid fold close to the nose is anchored lower down giving an oriental or 'Mongolian' appearance, a feature responsible

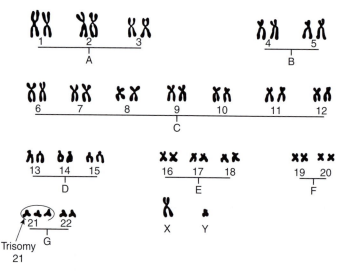

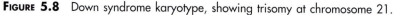

FIGURE 5.8 Down syndrome karyotype, showing trisomy at chromosome 21.

TABLE 5.2 Changes in the incidence to Down syndrome with maternal age

Maternal age at conception of child	Incidence of Down syndrome
Less than 30 years old	1 in 3000 live births
35 to 39 years old	1 in 280 live births
40 to 44 years old	1 in 70 live births
45 to 49 years old	1 in 40 live births

for the term *mongolism* which is sometimes inappropriately used). Other features are a large, furrowed tongue in a small mouth, a single crease in the palm of the hand (known as a **simian crease**) and a long plantar crease down the sole of the foot extending from an enlarged gap between the first two toes. There may also be increased extensibility of the limbs due to poor muscle tone. Varying degrees of congenital heart defects can occur, and cataracts (opacity of the lens of the eye causing blindness), squints and nystagmus (rapid uncontrollable lateral eye movements) are more common than in the average person.

The mental retardation can be anything from very mild to quite severe (Kaplan and Sadock 1996). At the mild end of the spectrum, Down syndrome children communicate and learn quite well and become relatively independent adults. They can perform quite intricate tasks and cope with jobs that are not too demanding. They are often happy and enjoy participating in activities such as learning a musical instrument, singing and dancing. Before the advent of modern social conditions and life-saving treatments such as antibiotics, Down syndrome children often died from neglect, undernutrition and infections. Now, many are living into adulthood, when they begin to face another problem. The middle aged Down syndrome adult (i.e. 30 to 40 years of age) often shows evidence of dementia of the type related to Alzheimer disease. Chapter 12 explores Alzheimer disease in some detail, and the connection with chromosome 21, relating this to Down syndrome.

See page 254

Deletions

In addition to extra chromosomes, chromosomal deletions may affect mental development. This type of mutation involves the loss of a genetic sequence, i.e. a number of DNA bases, often due to breakages during cell division.

Cri-du-chat (cry of cat) syndrome

This disorder involves the deletion of part of the short arm of chromosome 5 (Faraone *et al.* 1999). The specific gene locus involved is 5p15.2. This gene codes for **catenin delta-2**, a protein that is specific to neurons and is involved significantly in neural motility during the very early stages of nervous system development. Children born with this condition show mental retardation and severe physical abnormalities such as microcephaly (small head and brain), low-set ears and oblique palpebral fissures (openings of the eye). The disorder gets its name from a cat-like crying sound they make, but this gradually disappears as they get older.

Williams syndrome

This disorder is caused by the loss of a small fragment of genetic material from one of the 7th chromosomes, a loss of about 15 or so genes at 7q11.23. The other 7th chromosome is present and complete. The incidence of this condition is about one in every 20 000 births worldwide. It causes a minor degree of mental retardation, resulting in lower than average intelligence test scores. The surprise, however, is the remarkable musical talent that many with the disorder display. Williams syndrome people can often perform, remember and even compose music to a very high degree of competency (Lenhoff *et al.* 1997). Several genes that are missing from the deleted segment are involved in brain development, but their mechanism of action is not fully known.

The musical ability can be partly explained by studies of the brains from Williams syndrome people that show an extensive expansion of part of the temporal cortex called the **planum temporale**. This expansion is also found in gifted musicians without this syndrome (see music). However, other areas of the brain in Williams syndrome are reduced to below normal size.

See page 144

Prader–Willi and Angelman syndromes

Both these syndromes are caused by deletion of part of chromosome 15, i.e. the gene locus 15q11. The deletion in Prader–Willi syndrome appears to be

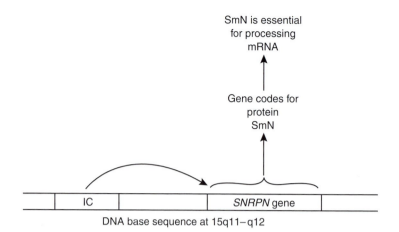

FIGURE 5.9 Angelman and Prader–Willi syndromes. The gene (*SRPN*) located at 15q11–q12 is controlled by an imprinting centre (IC) further along the DNA sequence. The gene codes for the SmN protein, which is important in processing mRNA. Mutations in the IC affect protein production, and this error is passed on to the offspring, through successive generations, from either the maternal line (Angelman) or paternal line (Prader–Willi).

limited to 15q11, while in Angelman syndrome the deletion is wider, to include 15q11 and 15q12, and sometimes part of 15q13. It appears that the difference depends on which parent the deletion was obtained from. If the deletion is inherited from the mother (the maternal line of inheritance), the resulting **syndrome** in the offspring is Angelman; if from the father (the paternal line of inheritance) it is Prader–Willi. This is possible because of a molecular process called **imprinting**. Imprinting is the process of switching a gene *on* (activation) or *off* (deactivation) by control from a genetic **imprinting centre** (**IC**), found a short distance along the genetic base sequence from the gene being controlled (Figure 5.9). At 15q11–q12 there is a gene called *SNRPN* (**small nuclear ribonucleoprotein N**), controlled by a nearby IC. *SNRPN* codes for a protein called **SmN** (a small nuclear ribonucleoprotein subunit), which is involved in the processing of **messenger ribonucleic acid** (**mRNA**), the molecule required to carry the DNA code to the ribosome for protein synthesis. SmN is particularly expressed in the brain. Disturbance in the activation of this gene could be a cause of inappropriate protein synthesis in specific neurons, leading to abnormal development of the brain or malfunction of those neurons. Mutations in the form of deletions in the IC of this gene appear to result in the fixing of the gene activation on a single parental line only. The deletions are probably due to the fact that this particular DNA sequence has two points that are susceptible to breakage.

Angelman syndrome is characterised by severe motor impairment, e.g. **ataxia** (poor coordination of movement and loss of balance), **hypotonia** (loose, floppy muscles), and mental retardation, including failure of speech and epilepsy. Other abnormal characteristics include a large mandible, which may protrude forward (**prognathism**), a large open mouth (**macrostomia**) with protruding tongue, excessive laughter (appears happy), puppet-like movements and hyperactivity.

Prader–Willi syndrome also shows symptoms of hypotonia and mental retardation. In this syndrome the sufferer develops a **hyperphagia**, i.e. an excessive appetite, which leads to overeating and obesity. People with this condition have small hands, small feet and a short stature, coupled with reduced levels of gonad function (**hypogonadism**) due to undersecretion of **gonadotrophic** hormones from the pituitary gland. Children may show defiant behaviour.

Both syndromes are rare; Prader–Willi syndrome, for example, affects fewer than one person in 10 000 (Kaplan and Sadock 1996).

The lissencephalic disorders

Lissencephaly ('**lissos**' = smooth, '**encephalon**' = brain; i.e. the 'smooth brain' disorders) includes a number **microdeletions** (very small genetic deletions), which result in a degree of mental retardation and other symptoms (Pilz and Quarrell 1996). In these disorders, abnormal neuronal migration occurs during fetal development, resulting in a smooth cortex, i.e. a significant loss of the normal folding into sulci and gyri, together with varying changes of cortical cell layers. Neuronal migration is described in Chapter 8. A gene that is vital in the control of cortical cell structure, *See page 168* called the **lissencephaly gene** (*LIS1*), has been discovered on chromosome 17. This gene is probably involved in cell signalling during fetal neuronal migration of the cerebrum. The microdeletion of this gene is a major cause of these 'smooth brain' disorders. Lissencephalic disorders are usually divided into **type I** ('**classical**'), and **type II** (**variant** or **Walker's lissencephaly**).

- Type I lissencephaly shows a smoothing of the brain surface with disruption of the cell structure (**cytoarchitecture**) causing a thick, four-layered cerebral cortex (normally, the cerebral cortex has six distinct cell layers). The cerebellum is basically normal. The clinical features are mental retardation, diplegia (bilateral paralysis) and fits. Type I lissencephaly is more likely to be sporadic in origin, rather than inherited. Sporadic genetic changes involve the affected individual only and are not passed on to subsequent generations through the sperm or ova. **Miller–Dieker syndrome** (**MDS**), which is caused by a microdeletion at gene locus 17p13.3, results in severe mental retardation with other neurological deficits (e.g. difficulty in swallowing), and growth deficiency with **craniofacial defects** (sometimes called the '**Miller–Dieker face**') involving a prominent forehead, a short, upturned nose, protruding upper lip and small jaw. Death usually occurs within the first year of life.
- Type II lissencephaly shows a smoothing of the brain surface with disruption of the cytoarchitecture in a manner that results in no distinct cell layers. The main features of type II are severe neurological dysfunction from an early age, eye abnormalities and hydrocephalus. Type *See page 88* II lissencephaly is thought more likely to be genetically inherited than

type I. The disorders that fall into the type II category are those that cause various forms of muscular dystrophy (muscle wasting with weakness) due to the neurological dysfunction. **Walker–Warburg syndrome** (**WWS**) is part of this group of muscle disorders known as the **congenital muscular dystrophies** (**CMD**), where muscle weakness, losses of muscle tone and muscle contractures are predominant symptoms (Leyten *et al.* 1996). It should not be surprising that a brain lissencephaly causes muscle problems since the main motor cortex that controls skeletal muscle movement is part of the cerebrum (Brodmann 4). Walker–Warburg syndrome, a cause of severe mental and psychomotor retardation, shows an autosomal recessive inheritance pattern, although it is not yet clear which chromosome and genes are involved.

See page 5

A deletion close to that seen in Miller–Dieker syndrome occurs at 17p11.2, resulting in the **Smith–Magenis syndrome**. This causes brachycephaly (short, broad skull caused by early closure of the coronal skull suture and excessive lateral skull growth), a prominent forehead, a broad face and nasal bridge, heart defects, hyperactivity and fits. Maladaptive behaviour causes problems such as self-harm and sleep pattern disturbance (Dykens and Smith 1998).

Genetic disorders

Apart from whole chromosomes or parts of chromosomes, a single gene or a few genes may be responsible for specific disorders involving mental health disturbance.

Learning and developmental disorders

The learning and developmental disorders are included here since most are considered to have a genetic basis as well as environmental factors involved in the causation, i.e. a polygenic aetiology. Where the actual genes of some conditions are unknown, the genetic hypothesis is based on hereditary patterns.

Autism

This condition is so called because affected children appear to withdraw from normal social interactions, including parental relations, and prefer their own company in isolation (auto = self). They fail to develop the skills necessary for normal human interactions; notably, communication skills are lacking to varying degrees or even absent. The social isolationism is akin to that seen in schizophrenia, a disorder to which autism is linked. Autism is also sometimes associated with other conditions, notably epilepsy, Rett's syndrome, Down syndrome, various single-gene defects, infections (e.g. congenital **rubella**, or German measles), some temporal lobe tumours and **hydrocephalus** (Rapin 1998). Hydrocephalus is excessive water around the brain due to a build-up of **cerebrospinal fluid** (**CSF**), which can cause

See page 167

See page 90
See page 83

extensive brain damage. The cause of autism therefore appears to be multifactorial, not purely genetic. The condition affects about 1 in 250 000 infants (0.0004%), with boys being more often affected than girls. There is now, however, compelling evidence that at least some forms of autism are genetically inherited. Twin studies offer the best evidence of this. If one **monozygotic (identical) twin** has autism, the other twin has up to 96% chance of having autism; that is, there is a **concordance rate** of 96%. In a case of concordance, both twins will develop the disorder, while in a case of **discordance**, one will but the other will not develop the disorder. In **dizygotic (nonidentical) twins** the concordance rate is about the same as for ordinary siblings with the disorder (i.e. 2–3%). Even 2% is a very much higher chance of developing the disorder than the 0.0004% recorded for the population as a whole, indicating that the figures for twins and sibling relationships is strongly influenced by inherited genetic factors. The genes themselves appear elusive, although a few genes and chromosomes are looking like strong candidates:

- a gene at locus 7q31, involved in speech, called *SPCH1*;
- deletion or **duplication** (repeated DNA sequences) of a gene on 15q11–13 (Folstein *et al.* 1998).

Genetic research has been centred on chromosomes 7 and 15 as these suspect genes are sequenced and their proteins are analysed. As a result, more information is likely to become available over the coming years.

Another important factor in autism is damage to the central nervous system of the fetus during or shortly after pregnancy. The highest incidence of autism occurs if fetal brain development is disturbed during the early stages of pregnancy.

In autism the brain shows evidence of abnormalities to the temporal lobe, cerebellum and the brain stem. Studies involving the biochemistry of the **prefrontal cortex** in males suffering from autism indicate disordered levels of the energy-related molecules, including reduced levels of **phosphocreatinine (PCr)**, suggesting that a hypermetabolic state exists in neurons of the frontal lobes with a lack of synthesis of cell membranes (Maier 1998). The **cerebellum** in autistic sufferers is also affected, showing a poorly developed **vermis** (Figure 5.10). The cerebellar vermis is a median lobe (that is, it runs along the midline) that appears worm-like (vermis = worm). The cerebellar vermis is also poorly developed, and sometimes missing, in an autosomal recessive disorder called **Joubert syndrome**. Children with this condition also show symptoms of autism, suggesting cerebellar involvement in the cause of some aspects of autism.

Autism in both children and adults often presents great challenges for nurses, parents and other carers at home. The principal problems centre around communication difficulties, and specialist advice and support are often required (Aylott 2000a, b). Part of the management of autism may be diet based. Some affected children have been found to benefit from the exclusion from the diet of both gluten (a wheat-based protein) and casein (a milk-based protein) (Miller 1995). The theory suggests that when these

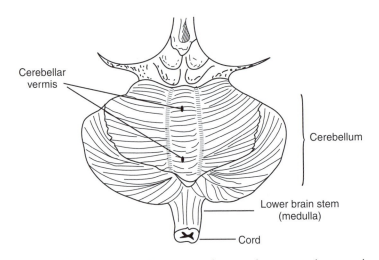

Cerebellar vermis

Cerebellum

Lower brain stem (medulla)

Cord

FIGURE 5.10 The cerebellum, dorsal view showing the vermis (the central ridge), malformation of which is becoming important in mental health.

peptides (small proteins) are absorbed they inhibit brain activity to some extent. Their removal from the diet is thought to give the brain greater potential to interact with the environment, improving the ability to talk and reducing the autistic traits. Dietary management is not a cure but it may help to improve the child's communication skills and increase interaction with the family.

Some individuals are considered to have a milder form of autism called **Asperger disorder** (or **Asperger syndrome**), named after Hans Asperger, an Austrian physician. They demonstrate varying degrees of the following symptoms:

- an inability to respond to normal social interactions with other people;
- restricted interests and behavioural patterns;
- inability to form peer relationships;
- poor reciprocal emotional abilities;
- abnormal nonverbal gestures.

This behaviour tends towards the isolationism also seen in autism, but in Asperger verbal communication and cognitive development are normal (Kaplan and Sadock 1996).

Rett syndrome

This is another condition that involves the clinical symptoms of autism. The sufferers, almost entirely girls, develop normally for about the first few months of life, then further development is arrested at about 12–18 months of age, followed by a serious decline in growth and development. This rapid decline includes autistic symptoms with dementia, and these may be the first clinical signs of this disorder. However, the genetic basis of the disease indicates that the syndrome is present from birth. The symptoms progress to include motor problems such as abnormal hand movements and failure to walk, failure of head growth leading to **microcephaly** (= small head) and in some cases a slight increase in the level of ammonia in the blood (**hyperammonaemia**). The gene most likely to be involved appears to be on the X chromosome; called *SYN1*, it codes for the protein **synapsin I**. This protein is one of several synapsins critically involved in **synaptogenesis** (the formation of synapses) and in the modulation of neurotransmitter release at the synapse. Exactly how the gene mutation causes the symptoms is not yet clear, but neuronal developmental problems have been found on brain examination. Brain cells show membrane-bound **inclusions** (abnormal structures within the cell body) in both neurons and oligodendrocytes, and a loss of dendrites from neurons extending from the motor and limbic cortex has also been identified.

Attention deficit disorder (ADD) and attention deficit hyperactive disorder (ADHD)

These two related conditions affect learning by disrupting the child's ability to raise attention and concentrate on any specific subject. The difference between them is the degree of additional hyperactive disruptive behaviour, which becomes a dominant feature of the condition in ADHD.

The symptoms of ADHD include severe impulsive, disruptive and aggressive behaviour, restlessness and inability to concentrate on a subject. Approximately 3% of the population suffer from this condition. The cause and the associated pathology are not fully understood, but recently there have been some interesting test results suggesting that these children lack some of the systems in the brain that inhibit impulsive and aggressive behaviour (Taylor 1999). Such an inability to block disruptive behaviour would result in acting without thinking or realising the consequences.

ADHD shows an autosomal dominant inheritance pattern with familial tendencies, although the genes and the mutations involved are still under investigation. It is often inherited along with other conditions which further complicate the picture. ADHD is regularly associated with substance abuse, for example alcoholism, and with depression. One gene in particular, found at locus 5p15.3, is strongly implicated in the condition. Called *DAT1*, this gene codes for a protein that transports the neurotransmitter dopamine across the cell membrane, but it not clear how this is involved in the condition. The brains of sufferers show little difference from the brains of normal controls, except for an 8% reduction in glucose metabolism in the premotor cortex and prefrontal cortex (both parts of the frontal lobe of the cerebrum). The treatment of ADHD may include prescription of the drug **methylphenidate hydrochloride (Ritalin)**. Related to amphetamines, it stimulates *See page 120* the central nervous system with increasing levels of dopamine, improving alertness and concentration. The drug remains controversial because it can produce side-effects such as nervousness, loss of appetite, insomnia, headaches, dizziness and, rarely, hallucinations. It can also affect the rest of the body, causing possible growth failure, damage to heart muscles and low blood cell counts. Some parents of affected children taking Ritalin have claimed remarkable transformations in their children in terms of better behaviour and concentration. However, other parents have said that this drug has not been beneficial, causing additional behavioural problems. In either case, there is clearly a need for a comprehensive treatment plan for all sufferers from ADHD, in which Ritalin may or may not form part of the therapy, based on a joint decision between medical staff and parents (Scott 2000).

Gilles de la Tourette syndrome (or Tourette syndrome)

This neurological disorder is characterised by motor and vocal **tics**, i.e. uncontrollable and repetitive muscle twitches of the head and shoulders particularly, and involuntary abnormal vocal sounds (e.g. grunts, barks, whistles). These tics are associated with abnormal behaviour, such as pulling hair and self-mutilation, and especially the compulsion to utter obscene words (**coprolalia**) and to repeat words many times (**echolalia**). The symptoms of the condition begin between the ages of 2 and 15 years and about 75% of the patients are male. There may be several genes involved in the aetiology of this disorder, with special emphasis placed on genes at the loci 11q23, 18q22.1 and 7q31. While some researchers propose one or another of these loci, others are unable to replicate the same findings, so the genetic hunt continues. The pathology of the brain in Tourette's syndrome appears to be centred on the dopaminergic systems of the basal ganglia. Dopamine receptor antagonists, particularly D_2 antagonists such as **haloperidol**, have reduced symptoms significantly, while drugs with a dopamimetic action (i.e. mimicking dopamine) make the symptoms worse. The basal ganglia is implicated in the disease because of its motor function and because some discrepancy in the symmetry of both the putamen and the lentiform nucleus has been identified in some sufferers (Rosenzweig et al. 1999). The putamen and the lentiform nucleus are both components of the basal ganglia.

See page 11

Dyslexia

Dyslexia is a reading disorder in which any three of the following symptoms may be present:

1 words or letters being reversed during reading after the age of 8 years;
2 deterioration of writing;
3 difficulty with hearing;
4 difficulty with learning by rote.

Between 5% and 10% of school children have significant deficits in their reading skills. Reading begins with the understanding of the phonics (or sounds) of words, or different parts of words, learnt first from the spoken language. After this, the child must learn to associate the phonic sounds with the written symbols of the language as printed on the page, so reading becomes a translation of the written symbols into spoken sounds. Sufferers of dyslexia appear to find this very difficult, although in all other respects they may be intellectually well developed. Developmental dyslexia appears to be familial, suggesting a genetic basis to the disorder.

Three genes have been identified as associated with dyslexia:

- **DYX1** (dyslexia specific 1) coded at 15q21, a gene linked to single-word reading and spelling. Disorder of this gene results in both spelling and reading difficulties, providing a biological basis that accounts for the linkage between these two skills.
- **DYX2** (dyslexia specific 2) coded at 6p21.3, a gene linked to the awareness of phonics in the spoken word.
- **DYX3** (dyslexia specific 3) a recently discovered gene of which little is currently known.

Investigations into the brains of sufferers of dyslexia have identified disorganised cell layers within part of the thalamus, the **lateral geniculate nucleus (LGN)**, which is the relay point for visual stimuli from the retina of the eye to the visual cortex within the occipital lobe of the cerebrum. The thalamic cells that are disrupted are those of the **magnocellular layers** (Figure 5.11), large cells that convey sensory impulses relating to visual depth of field and the visual perception of movement to the visual cortex. Other thalamic cells within the LGN, the **parvocellular layers**, which convey colour and fine detail impulses to the cortex, are unaffected by the disorder. Pathways from the magnocellular layers of the LGN activate the part of the visual cortex called V5, which functions in the event of movement within the visual field. In dyslexia, V5 activation by the sensory input from the LGN magnocellular layers appears not to happen. Reading is affected, possibly because words appear to the reader to move around on

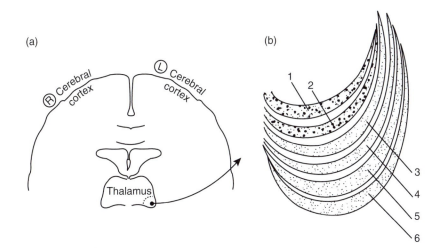

Figure 5.11 The magnocellular layer (layers 1 and 2) of the lateral geniculate nucleus of the thalamus, which are disrupted in dyslexia. Layers 3 to 6, the parvonuclear layers, are unaffected.

the page and become jumbled, and this is a common complaint made by sufferers of dyslexia. They transpose letters within a word and this causes them to misread words; for example, the written word *dog* is read as *god*. Perhaps the magnocellular layers are distorting the visual image of words and may be adding unnecessary movement, possibly in relation to the movement of the eyes themselves. Movement involves space, and other symptoms associated with dyslexia show disturbance to movement and space-related skills including poor handwriting, difficulties with balance (e.g. when riding a bicycle), delayed walking skills and slowness in learning how to tell the time. These skills require visual input and the difficulties found in dyslexia suggest problems associated with the development of the posterior parietal lobe, i.e. the primary visual cortex, or its input from the visual pathways via the LGN (Carlson 2001).

Dyslexic people also seem to have part of their upper temporal lobe, the **planum temporale**, equal in size on both sides. Normally, the left planum temporale is larger than the right (Figure 5.12). Only 11% of the population have a right planum temporale larger than the left. The fact that they are

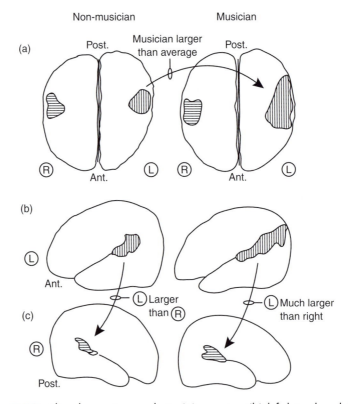

FIGURE 5.12 The planum temporale in (a) superior, (b) left lateral and (c) right lateral views. Normally, the left planum temporale is larger than the right in most people. In musicians, especially those with perfect pitch, the left planum temporale is considerably larger than the right. In those with dyslexia the planum temporale tends to be of equal size on both sides.

more or less symmetrical in dyslexia is significant. This region contains **Wernicke's area,** the language area, and this has led to speculation that the planum temporale is normally larger and more dominant on the left because it is involved in language and speech perception. Whether this is true or not is a debate that continues.

Dysgraphia

Dysgraphia is a disorder of writing, causing problems with spelling, in two main forms:

- **Phonological dysgraphia,** the inability to write words phonetically, or according to the sounds of words. This disorder is thought to be caused by neuronal damage to the superior temporal lobe. The ability to write whole words is retained.
- **Orthographic dysgraphia,** the inability to write and spell visually based irregular words. Thus the ability to write whole words is poor, whilst phonetic writing is preserved. This disorder is thought to be caused by neuronal damage to the inferior parietal lobe.

Writing is a function primarily of that half of the brain dominant for speech, the left hemisphere of the cerebral cortex in most people. It is here that the twin speech areas are located, **Wernicke's area** for language construction and **Broca's** area for the motor organisation of the muscles for speech.

Dyspraxia

Dyspraxia is a disorder of movement in which specific motor skills cannot be carried out despite there being no evidence of paralysis. It is the speed of movements that appears to be impeded. Speech is affected in some cases (**verbal dyspraxia**) because speech involves rapid, skilled movements of the jaw and tongue. In normal speech we are capable of producing as many as 15 sounds every second. Sufferers of dyspraxia may also have some degree of difficulty with reading (an overlap with dyslexia) or with purposeful movements, thus appearing clumsy (sometimes called **motor dyspraxia**). Swallowing and sucking movements remain normal.

Sex chromosomes

The genetic determination of an individual's sex relies on the inheritance of a combination of the **sex chromosomes**, **X** and **Y**. The **XX** combination produces a female and the **XY** combination produces a male. 'Maleness' therefore requires the presence of the Y chromosome, while 'femaleness' requires the absence of the Y chromosome.

Several genes are involved in creating the male condition, one of which is very close to the **centromere** on the Y chromosome (Figure 5.13). This is the *SRY* **gene** (i.e. the **sex-determining region Y**), a gene that codes for

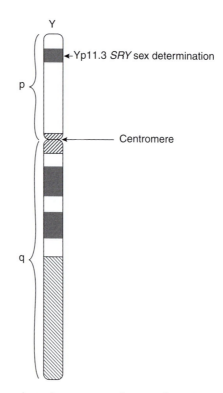

Y

←Yp11.3 *SRY* sex determination

p

———— Centromere

q

FIGURE 5.13 The male Y chromosome, showing the *SRY* (sex determination) gene locus at Yp11.3.

a **transcription factor**. Transcription factors are proteins that bind to DNA and begin to trigger the process of RNA assembly, the process called **transcription**, leading to protein synthesis.

The *SRY*-encoded transcription factor switches on testicular development in the primitive gonad, which up to that point has been undifferentiated, being neither testes nor ovary. In addition, it has been found that *SRY* genes are also expressed in parts of the male mouse brain, notably the hypothalamus and the midbrain, suggesting that a similar expression in male human brains may trigger sex-determination within these brain structures (Lahr *et al.* 1995). H-Y antigen is another factor that predisposes towards the male condition, by promoting testicular development in the primitive, undifferentiated gonads. The gene that codes for the structure of H-Y antigen is on an **autosome** (chromosome 6), but its expression is suppressed (or inhibited) by factors coded on the X chromosome. Other Y chromosome factors block the X chromosome factors, a case of inhibiting the inhibitor, and this allows the expression of the H-Y antigen (Figure 5.14). There is about 1000 times more male H-Y antigen than female H-Y antigen due to the Y inhibition of the X factor in males (Lau *et al.* 1986, 1987).

XXY males are described as having **Klinefelter syndrome** (Figure 5.15). The additional X chromosome changes the normal karyotype of 46 chromosomes into the abnormal number of 47. Klinefelter syndrome

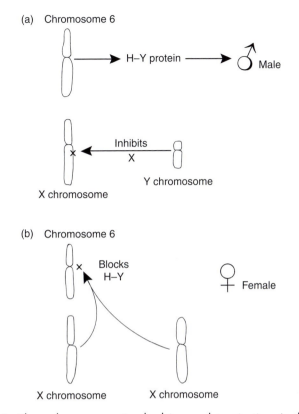

(a) Chromosome 6

(b) Chromosome 6

FIGURE 5.14 Three chromosomes involved in sex determination. In the male (a), chromosome 6 has the gene for the H–Y protein that causes masculinisation. The presence of a Y chromosome produces an inhibiting factor that blocks the X chromosome. In the female (b), the absence of a Y chromosome allows both X chromosomes to block the H–Y protein from chromosome 6, and the female condition will develop.

is the result of fertilisation involving either **diploid sperm** or **diploid ova**. Diploid in this context means that the sperm or ovum carries *both* the sex chromosomes instead of just one; thus one ovum would carry XX, or one sperm would carry XY. On fertilisation with a normal Y sperm, the XX ovum would become XXY. Fertilisation between an XY sperm and a normal X ovum would also result in XXY (see Figure 5.16). Klinefelter syndrome occurs in 1 in 600 live births and, because the Y is present, the child is always male. However, males with this condition are usually tall, often thin, with poor sexual development and are mildly mentally retarded. It would appear that the more extra X chromosomes present, the greater is the degree of mental retardation (McCance and Huether 1994; Woolfe 1998).

Figure 5.15 also shows an XXX combination, which is the inappropriately named **superwoman syndrome**. This is another 47-chromosome karyotype, caused by a **trisomy X**. As for the male in Klinefelter syndrome, the XXX female sometimes has poor sexual development and a mild mental retardation. Superwoman syndrome is rarer than Klinefelter syndrome, occurring in 1 in 1600 live births. In both cases the additional X causes mild mental

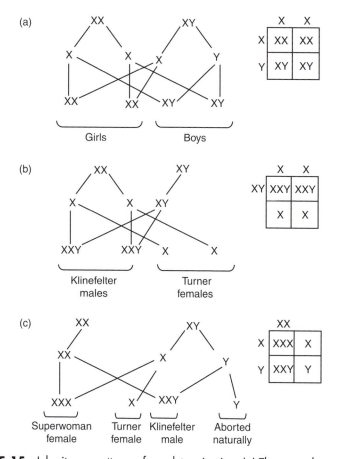

FIGURE 5.15 Inheritance patterns of sex determination. (a) The normal cross-over of the female XX and male XY to produce a 50% chance of either sex. (b) Abnormal male clustering together of the XY chromosomes, giving sons with Klinefelter syndrome, or daughters with Turner's syndrome. (c) Abnormal female clustering together of the XX chromosomes, giving sons that either are Klinefelter syndrome or are incompatible with life and will spontaneously abort, or giving daughters who may be superwoman syndrome or Turner's syndrome. All three are shown as cross-overs or punnet squares.

retardation, but people with these syndromes are able to live normally in society. This is not so true for the very rare cases of XXXY or XXXX syndromes reported, where more X chromosomes cause greater degrees of mental retardation. Curfs *et al.* (1990) described several XXXXY male patients with moderate to profound mental retardation and emotional disturbances.

As shown in Figure 5.15, the single X (**monosomy X**) female also occurs, giving a 45-chromosome karyotype. Monosomy X is **Turner's syndrome**, characterised by a short female with poor sexual development and some minor physical abnormalities. However, with one X present these females

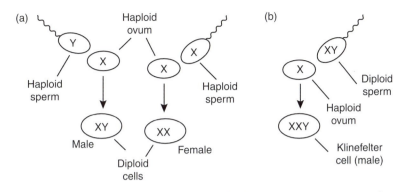

FIGURE 5.16 Sperm meets ovum. (a) Normally the sperm carries one sex chromosome (either X or Y) and this meets the ovum that carries one X chromosome to produce a fertilised ovum with XX or XY. (b) Sometimes an abnormal sperm carries both XY and meets a normal ovum to give a fertilised ovum with XXY. Normal sperm fertilising abnormal XX ovum to give either XXX or XXY also occurs occasionally (not shown).

have normal mental development. Turner's syndrome happens in about 1 in 3000 live births.

XYY males do occur as well, since nearly 1% of all sperm carry the YY chromosome combination which may fertilise a normal single X ovum to cause XYY. It perhaps happens in 1 in 1000 live births. These males have attracted a great deal of research because this particular genetic combination was quite early associated with aggression and criminal behaviour. The XYY combination was first reported in 1961 and its association with violent criminal behaviour was made in 1965. Today, much of this original work on XYY is seen to be inappropriate and flawed because of sample bias, since most of the work focused on male prison populations. We now know that less than 1% of all XYY men become prisoners and that less than 2% of male prisoners are XYY. Leaving prison populations aside, XYY may cause some small increase in antisocial behaviour when compared to the normal XY or even XXY combinations. Other characteristics of the XYY male include above-average height, around 73 inches compared to the XY average of 67 inches. Even as a child of 6 years, the XYY male is taller than 90% of his peers of the same age. Sexual development is normal, but there will be poor coordination, delayed language skills and some learning difficulties. These males generally perform less well in intelligence quotient (IQ) tests than their XY counterparts, approximately on a par with XXY males.

Very rarely, XYYY and even XYYYY males have been reported, but unlike the additional X chromosomes, the additional Ys have little or no effect on mental development.

The X chromosome is much larger than the Y chromosome and this means that it carries many more genes. It is the source of significantly large numbers of rare but important mental retardation syndromes (Figure 5.17). The mental health nurse, who is in the best position to encounter

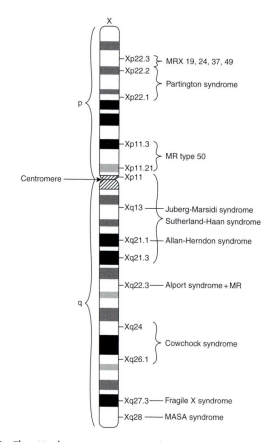

FIGURE 5.17 The X chromosome. Several important mental retardation (MR) syndromes are located on both the p (short) and q (long) arms.

them, should be aware of these syndromes. Table 5.3 lists the better-known X-linked syndromes that result in some degree of mental retardation and also illustrates the large number of mental retardation syndromes associated with the X chromosome. Notice in Figure 5.17 that there are a number of mental retardation syndromes positioned in clusters on the chromosome, the **loci** of the major ones being Xp22.3–p22.2; Xp11.3–p11.21 (close to the centromere); Xq21.3–q24 and Xq28.

The term **phenotype** refers to the physical features caused by the **genotype**, or genes present in the cell. Another way of stating this is to say that the genotype consists of the genes locked up in the cell nucleus, while the phenotype is the bodily features (tall, short, etc.), created by expression of the genes. Other terms included in Table 5.3 are **adducted thumbs**, where the thumbs lie closer to the hand than normally; **aphasia**, the inability to speak; **brachycephaly**, a congenital skull malformation in which the head is short but wide; **dysarthria**, a difficulty with speech due to poor speech muscle control; **dystonic (dystonia)**, an abnormal posture of a limb or the trunk with slow and twisting movements; **elliptocytosis**, a mild increase in the numbers of elliptocytes (oval instead of round erythrocytes) such that

TABLE 5.3 X-linked syndromes involving mental retardation

Gene locus	Syndrome name or code (if any)	Phenotype	Reference
Xp22.3–22.2	MRX19, 24, 37		Claes *et al.* (1997)
Xp22.3–22.2	MRX49	Mild to moderate MR	Claes *et al.* (1997)
Xp22.3–21.3		MR in males only	Hane *et al.* (1996)
Xp22.2–p22.1	Partington syndrome	Male only, mild to moderate MR, dystonic hand movements, dysarthria	Partington *et al.* (1988)
Xp21–q13		Varying degree of MR	Willems *et al.* (1993)
Xp11–q21.3	Sutherland–Haan X-linked MR syndrome	Short stature, small testes, microcephaly, brachycephaly, MR	
Xp11.3–p11.21	MR type 50	Moderate MR	Claes *et al.* (1997)
Xq13	Juberg–Marsidi syndrome	Probably males only. Growth delay, facial anomalies, deafness, MR and microgenitalism	Juberg and Marsidi (1980)
Xq21.1	Allan–Herndon syndrome	Severe MR, muscle and movement anomalies, head abnormalities	Allan *et al.* (1944)
Xq22		Female epilepsy + MR	Juberg and Hellman (1971)
Xq22.3		Alport syndrome (multiple physical deformities and disorders, worse in males) with MR, elliptocytosis, midface hypoplasia	Jonsson *et al.* (1998)
Xq24–26.1	Cowchock syndrome	Neuropathy, deafness and MR. Worse in males	Cowchock *et al.* (1985)
Xq26–27		Male moderate MR + facial abnormalities and large testes	Shashi *et al.* (2000)
Xq27.3	Fragile X syndrome	See text	
Xq28	MASA syndrome	MR, aphasia, shuffling gait, adducted thumbs	Bianchine and Lewis (1974)
X	Chudley MR syndrome	Moderate to severe MR, short stature, mild obesity, hypogonadism, facial abnormalities	Chudley *et al.* (1988)

MR = mental retardation. X = X chromosome (MRX with a number refers to a specific mental retardation syndrome). p = short arm. q = long arm. See text for other definitions of terms. References are included to allow the interested student to seek further details.

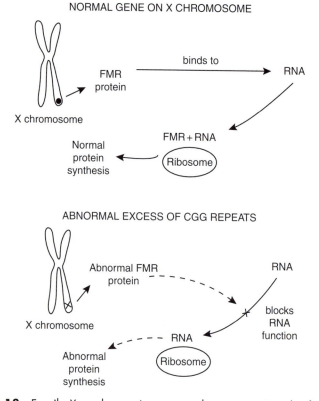

NORMAL GENE ON X CHROMOSOME

ABNORMAL EXCESS OF CGG REPEATS

FIGURE 5.18 Fragile X syndrome. A gene on chromosome X codes for the FMR protein, which appears to be important for RNA binding at the ribosome (top). In fragile X syndrome faulty DNA at the FMR gene causes failure of normal FMR protein which in turns reduces RNA's ability to bind at the ribosome (below). Failure of RNA binding reduces the cell's protein production ability, and the neuron will suffer from the loss.

the normal number of elliptocytes in the blood is less than 15%; **gait**, the method of walking; **hypogonadism**, underdevelopment of either testes or ovum; **hypoplasia**, reduced numbers of cells causing underdevelopment of an organ; and **microcephaly**, a small head with a small brain; **neuropathy**, disorder of the nerves.

Fragile X syndrome (Figure 5.18) is a mental retardation syndrome that illustrates an important point concerning the nature of genetic error. Fragile X is not the result of a simple mutation; it is caused by a **trinucleotide repeat**, where the same three genetic bases are repeated many times. The repeated bases are **CGG** (i.e. **cytosine–guanine–guanine**), where CGG codes for the amino acid **arginine**. Up to 54 such repeats occur normally, but any number of repeats from 52 to more than 200 are found in the syndrome. When expressed, the normal gene would code for a protein, known as the **FMR protein**, which binds with RNA (ribonucleic acid). RNA binding is critical at the ribosome where **translation** of the RNA code into a protein (protein synthesis) takes place. FMR has a number of characteristics required of a ribosomal protein. In fragile X syndrome, however, the CGG repeats block gene expression, with the consequent loss of the normal protein and a subsequent loss of RNA binding ability. This leads to failure of the cell's protein synthesis functions, and in neurons this causes varying degrees of mental retardation (Figure 5.18). Males appear to be more affected than females (only 30–40% of affected females have some degree of mental retardation). Less commonly, other symptoms occur, notably enlarged testes at puberty, large ears, a prominent jaw, some enlargement of the head in a few affected males, finger joints that extend farther than expected owing to loose connective tissues, and aortic and heart valve disorders. Speech may be delayed and high pitched. Trinucleotide repeats, which are also sometimes called **stuttering genes**, are of growing importance in mental health, and are implicated in other disorders such as **Huntington disease** and **schizophrenia**.

See page 232
See page 162

Key points

Chromosomes and genes

- Autosomes are chromosomes 1 to 22 in the human karyotype, 22 pairs of autosomes.
- Each pair consists of two chromosomes that are the same, called homologous chromosomes.
- Two alternative versions of the same gene are called alleles, one allele on each chromosome.
- Being from different parents, these alleles are of different traits.
- Whether a gene is expressed into the phenotype or not depends on whether it is dominant, recessive or co-dominant.
- Genes demonstrate varying degrees of penetrance, or how much each individual gene contributes to the completed body (the phenotype).
- The DNA determines what proteins will be produced, the amino acids it will contain and their sequence in the protein.
- Genes are found on the chromosome at sites called the gene locus (or slot), written by giving the chromosome number first, then the arm of the chromosome, 'p' for short arm and 'q' for long arm.
- Mutations are DNA errors, e.g. point mutations, translocations, deletions, frame shifts, inversions, base-sequence repeats and fragile sites.

Disorders of inheritance

- Inherited genetic disorders are often familial, i.e. found in successive generations of the same family.
- First-degree relatives of an affected person are their parents, brothers, sisters, sons or daughters; second-degree relatives are their grandparents, aunts or uncles; and third-degree relatives are those such as cousins.
- Monozygotic (MZ) twins are identical twins and share all their genes (i.e. all their genes are the same); dizygotic (DZ) twins are nonidentical twins and share about half of their genes.

Chromosomal disorders

- A genetic disorder may involve one gene or a few genes, but a chromosomal disorder involves abnormalities of whole or part of a chromosome, adding up to perhaps several thousand genes.
- A trisomy is one extra chromosome attached to a pair; a monosomy is only one chromosome instead of a pair.
- Trisomy 8 involves three number 8 chromosomes; trisomy 13 involves three number 13 chromosomes, called Patau syndrome; trisomy 18 involves three number 18 chromosomes, called Edward syndrome; and trisomy 21 involves three number 21 chromosomes, called Down syndrome.
- Cri-du-chat syndrome (cry of cat syndrome) is caused by a deletion of part of the short arm of chromosome 5.
- Prader–Willi and Angelman syndromes are both caused by deletion of part of chromosome 15 at the gene locus 15q11.
- If the deletion is inherited from the mother it causes Angelman syndrome, whilst it inherited from the father it causes Prader–Willi syndrome. This phenomenon is called imprinting, a process of switching a gene *on* or *off* in specific parental lines.
- Lissencephalies, the 'smooth brain' disorders, include a number microdeletions resulting in mental retardation and other symptoms. These disorders include Miller–Dieker and Walker–Warburg syndromes.

Learning and developmental disorders

- Good candidate genes for autism are at locus 7q31, a gene involved in speech called *SPCH1*, and on 15q.
- The prefrontal cortex in autism indicates disordered levels of the energy-related molecules, especially reduced levels of phosphocreatinine (PCr), suggesting that a hypermetabolic state exists in neurons of the frontal lobes.
- The cerebellum in autistic sufferers is also affected, showing a poorly developed vermis.
- A milder form of autism is called Asperger syndrome.
- Rett syndrome also involves the clinical picture of autism, the sufferers being almost always girls.
- The gene most likely involved in Rett syndrome is at locus Xp11.4–11.2, a gene called *SYN1* that codes for the protein synapsin I. Several synapsins occur, they are involved in synaptogenesis (the formation of synapses) and in the modulation of neurotransmitter release at the synapse.
- A gene called *DAT1*, found at locus 5p15.3, may be one factor causing attention deficit hyperactive disorder (ADHD). It codes for a protein that transports the neurotransmitter dopamine across the cell membrane.
- There may be several genes involved in the aetiology of Tourette syndrome, in particular 11q23, 18q22.1 and 7q.31.
- Two genes have been identified associated with dyslexia, *DYX1* (dyslexia specific 1) coded at 15q21, a gene linked to single word reading and

spelling, and *DYX2* (dyslexia specific 2) coded at 6p21.3, a gene linked to the awareness of phonics in the spoken word.

- The brains of dyslexia sufferers show disorganised cell layers within part of the thalamus, called the lateral geniculate nucleus (LGN), part of the visual pathway.
- Dysgraphia is a disorder of writing and spelling, in two forms: phonological dysgraphia and orthographic dysgraphia.

Sex chromosomes

- The sex chromosomes are X and Y, where XX corresponds to female and XY to male. 'Maleness' requires the Y chromosome, whilst 'femaleness' occurs in the absence of the Y chromosome.
- The normal karyotype contains 46 chromosomes.
- Abnormal karyotypes exist: an XXY male shows Klinefelter syndrome and an XXX individual shows superwoman syndrome. XYY males also occur. These conditions are all trisomies, where three chromosomes are in place of two (giving 47 chromosomes).
- Monosomy means one chromosome in place of two (giving 45 chromosomes). Monosomy X is Turner's syndrome.
- The X chromosome is the source of a large variety of mental retardation syndromes, albeit that they are generally rare.

References

Allan W., Herndon C. N. and Dudley F. C. (1944) Some examples of the inheritance of mental deficiency: apparently sex-linked idiocy and microcephaly. *American Journal of Mental Deficiency*, **48**: 325–334.

Aylott J. (2000a) Understanding children with autism: exploding the myths. *British Journal of Nursing*, **9** (12): 779–784.

Aylott J. (2000b) Autism in adulthood: the concepts of identity and difference. *British Journal of Nursing*, **9** (13): 851–858.

Bianchine J. W. and Lewis R. C., Jr. (1974) The MASA syndrome: a new heritable mental retardation syndrome. *Clinical Genetics*, **5**: 298–306.

Carlson N. R. (2001) *Physiology of Behavior*. Allyn and Bacon, Boston.

Chudley A. E., Lowry R. B. and Hoar D. I. (1988) Mental retardation, distinct facial changes, short stature, obesity, and hypogonadism: a new X-linked mental retardation syndrome. *American Journal of Medical Genetics*, **31**: 741–751.

Claes S., Vogels A., Holvoet M., Devriendt K., Raeymaekers P., Cassiman J. J. and Fryns J. P. (1997) Regional localisation of two genes for non-specific X-linked mental retardation to Xp22.3–p22.2 (MRX49) and Xp11.3–p11.21 (MRX50). *American Journal of Medical Genetics*, **73**: 474–479.

Cohen P. (2000) Shaping up. *New Scientist*, **165** (2227): 16.

Cowchock F. S., Duckett S. W., Streletz L. J., Graziani L. J. and Jackson L. G. (1985) X-linked motor-sensory neuropathy type-II with deafness and mental retardation: a new disorder. *American Journal of Medical Genetics*, **20**: 307–315.

Curfs L. M., Schrepers-Tijdink G., Wiegers A., Borghgraef M. and Fryns J. P. (1990) The 49, XXXXY syndrome: clinical and psychological findings in five patients. *Journal of Mental Deficiency Research*, **34** (3): 277–282.

Dykens E. M. and Smith A. C. M. (1998) Distinctiveness and correlates of maladaptive behaviour in children and adolescents with Smith–Magenis syndrome. *Journal of Intellectual Disability Research*, **42** (6): 481–489.

Faraone S. V., Tsuang M. T. and Tsuang D. W. (1999) *Genetics of Mental Disorder, a Guide for Students, Clinicians and Researchers*. The Guilford Press, London.

Folstein S. E., Haines J. and Santangelo S. L. (1998) The genetics of autism. *Neuroscience News* **1** (4): 14–17.

Hane B., Schroer R. J., Arena J. F., Lubs H. A., Schwartz C. E. and Stevenson R. E. (1996) Nonsyndromic X-linked mental retardation: review and mapping of MRX29 to Xp21. *Clinical Genetics*, **50**: 176–183.

Jonsson J. J., Renieri A., Gallagher P. G., Kashtan C. E., Cherniske E. M., Bruttini M., Piccini M., Vitelli F., Ballabio A. and Pober B. R. (1998) Alport syndrome, mental retardation, midface hypoplasia, and elliptocytosis: a new X-linked contiguous gene deletion syndrome. *Journal of Medical Genetics*, **35**: 273–278.

Juberg R. C. and Hellman C. D. (1971) A new familial form of convulsive disorder and mental retardation limited to females. *Journal of Pediatrics*, **79**: 726–732.

Juberg R. C. and Marsidi I. (1980) A new form of X-linked mental retardation with growth retardation, deafness and microgenitalism. *American Journal of Human Genetics*, **32**: 714–722.

Kaplan H. I. and Sadock B. J. (1996) *Concise Textbook of Clinical Psychiatry*. Williams and Wilkins, Baltimore.

Kimura D. (1992) Sex Differences in the Brain. http://www.scientificamerican.com/2002/0602mind/0602kimura.html

Lahr G., Maxson S. C., Mayer A., Just W., Pilgrim C. and Reisert I. (1995) Transcription of the Y chromosome gene, *Sry*, in adult mouse brain. *Brain Research Molecular Brain Research* **33** (1): 179–182.

Lau Y. F., Chan K., Kan Y. W. and Goldberg E. (1986) Isolation of a male-specific and conserved gene using an anti-H-Y antibody. *American Journal of Human Genetics*, **39**, A142.

Lau Y. F., Chan K., Kan Y. W. and Goldberg E. (1987) Structure and expression of a gene isolated with an anti-H-Y antibody, *Clinical Research*, **35**: 647A.

Lenhoff H. M., Wang P. P., Greenberg F. and Bellugi U. (1997) Williams syndrome and the brain. *Scientific American*, **277** (6): 42–47.

Leyten Q. H., Gabreels F. J. M., Renier W. O. and Ter Laak H. J. (1996) Congenital muscular dystrophy: a review of the literature. *Clinical Neurology and Neurosurgery*, **98** (4): 267–280.

McCance K. L. and Huether S. E. (1994) *Pathophysiology, The Biological Basis of Disease in Adults and Children*. Mosby, St Louis.

Maier M. (1998) Magnetic resonance spectroscopy in neuropsychiatry, *in* Ron M. A. and David A. S. (eds), *Disorders of Brain and Mind*, pp. 303–335. Cambridge University Press, Cambridge.

Miller K. (1995) Psychoneurological aspects of food allergy, *in* Leonard B. E. and Miller K. (eds), *Stress, the Immune System and Psychiatry*. Wiley, Chichester.

Partington M. W., Mulley J. C., Sutherland G. R., Hockey A., Thode A. and Turner G. (1988) X-linked mental retardation with dystonic movements of the hands. *American Journal of Medical Genetics*, **30**: 251–262.

Pilz D. T. and Quarrell O. W. J. (1996) Syndromes with lissencephaly. *Journal of Medical Genetics*, **33** (4): 319–323.

Rapin I. (1998) What a neurologist would like to know about autism and doesn't. *Neuroscience News*, **1** (4): 6–13.

Rosenzweig M. R., Leiman A. L. and Breedlove S. M. (1999) *Biological Psychology: An Introduction to Behavioural, Cognitive and Clinical Neuroscience*. Sinauer Associates, Sunderland, MA.

Scott S. (2000) Bad behaviour. *New Scientist*, **166** (2239): 44–45.

Shashi V., Berry M. N., Shoaf S., Sciote J. J., Goldstein D. and Hart T. C. (2000) A unique form of mental retardation with a distinctive phenotype maps to Xq26–q27. *American Journal of Human Genetics*, **66**: 469–479.

Taylor E. (1999) Early disorders and later schizophrenia: a developmental neuropsychiatric perspective, *in* Ron M. A. and David A. S. (eds) *Disorders of Brain and Mind*. Cambridge University Press, Cambridge.

Willems P., Vits L., Buntinx I., Raeymaekers P., Van Broeckhoven C., Ceulemans B. (1993) Localisation of a gene responsible for nonspecific mental retardation (MRX9) to the pericentromeric region of the X chromosome. *Genomics*, **18**: 290–294.

Woolfe N. (1998) *Pathology, Basic and Systemic*. W. B. Saunders, London.

Chapter 6

Drug use and abuse

Introduction to neuropharmacology

Pharmacodynamics

The study of the way drugs work is called **pharmacodynamics**. Understanding drug activity is important for both the prescribing and the delivery of drug treatment, and for making sense of side-effects.

Neuropharmacology (dealing with the drugs affecting the nervous system) involves two basic drug actions, the **agonist** and the **antagonist** (Figure 6.1). Agonist drugs bind to receptors and activate the receptor in a manner similar to that of the natural ligand (the neurotransmitter), and in

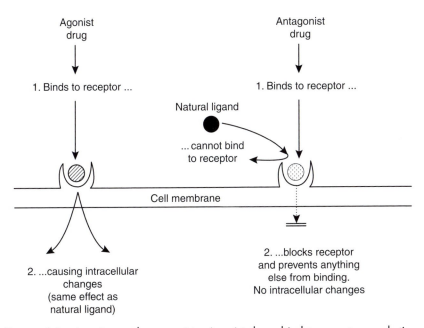

FIGURE 6.1 Agonists and antagonists. Agonist drugs bind to receptors and stimulate those receptors, causing the same effect as the natural ligand (the substance that binds naturally to the receptor). They therefore increase the effect of the receptor. Antagonists bind to the receptor but do not stimulate them. Instead, they block the receptor (often they are known as *blockers*), preventing the natural ligand from binding. They therefore reduce the effect of the receptor.

this way the drug enhances the neurotransmitter activity. Antagonist drugs also bind to receptors but do not activate them. Instead, they block the receptor, thus preventing the binding of the natural ligand and the stimulation of the receptor. Antagonists are often called *blockers* as an indication of their role in preventing receptor activation.

Other drugs work by influencing the levels of neurotransmitter produced at the synapse or by adjusting the sensitivity of the receptors. An increase in the production of neurotransmitter when levels are low can be achieved by drugs that either block the re-uptake of the ligand into the presynaptic bulb or inhibit the enzymes that metabolise the transmitter after use. The result is a greater amount of neurotransmitter in the synapse. Antidepressants work in one or other of these two ways. Some drugs modify the transmission of action potentials along the axon or at the cell body by preventing the influx of sodium or calcium through their channels. These drugs may be used in epilepsy to reduce the number and intensity of action potentials caused during a fit.

See page 194

Psychiatric drugs

Drugs used in psychiatry can be classified into eight main functional groups. Details of drug action can be found in the relevant chapters.

See page 53
1 **Sedatives**, which have a calming effect in low dosage, but can induce sleep in larger doses. These include the benzodiazepines, which bind to the GABA$_A$ receptor and enhance the action of GABA.

See page 155
2 **Anxiolytics**, which calm the mind without causing sleep. Of these, the benzodiazepines are important, but some are non-benzodiazepines.

See page 53
3 **Barbiturates**, which cause sleep or sedate the mind. Like benzodiazepines, these drugs bind to the GABA$_A$ receptor and enhance the action of GABA.

See page 173
4 **Antipsychotics**, which alter behaviour without causing sleep. They have a calming effect and reduce psychotic symptoms. Drugs of this group are dopamine receptor antagonists.

See page 198
5 **Antimanics**, mood-stabilising drugs, such as lithium.

6 **Antidepressants**, drugs that elevate mood by adjusting the sensitivity of serotonin and noradrenaline receptors as well as increasing the levels of these neurotransmitters in the synaptic cleft.

See page 194
7 **CNS stimulants**, used in the treatment of narcolepsy and attention deficit disorder. These work by increasing the levels of dopamine in the synaptic clefts of doperminergic neurons.

8 **Anticonvulsants**, which may be GABA$_A$ receptor-enhancing drugs, or sodium or calcium channel blockers, which prevent excessive action potentials.

See page 217

Pharmacokinetics

The study of drug movement in the body is called **pharmacokinetics**. Oral medication is affected by the processes of digestion, absorption, transportation by the blood, liver function, tissue storage and excretion (Kaplan and Sudock 1996). Digestive enzymes or stomach acidity may make some drugs unsuitable for administration by the oral route, and these may require injection. Absorption takes longer from the digestive tract than from a muscle, so medication administered intramuscularly acts more quickly than drugs taken by mouth. Oral drugs are first absorbed into the hepatic portal vein and thus are delivered to the liver first, where some breakdown of the drug occurs. This is called **first pass metabolism**, the liver effectively removing some of the dose before the drug enters the general circulation. Therefore, not all the oral dosage given becomes active drug in the body. Intramuscular administration is more efficient because the drug is absorbed from the muscle into the *systemic* capillaries first, then into the *systemic* veins, not the *hepatic portal* vein, so that the drug is not affected by first pass metabolism.

In the blood, drugs are usually bound to proteins, mostly **albumin**. Only unbound (or free) drug is available for use (known as the **bioavailability**) and the bound drug must be freed from the protein in order to increase its bioavailability before it enters the tissues. Some drugs bind to proteins or fat in the tissues and are then slowly released from there. This temporary 'storage' prolongs the time for which drugs are active in the body. The more fat there is in the tissues, the more the drug is bound up in this way, making

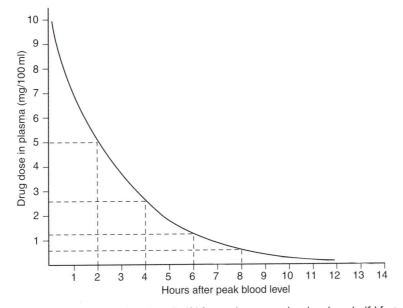

FIGURE 6.2 Illustration of a drug half-life. In this example, the drug half-life is 2 hours. By 2 hours after peak blood level, metabolism has removed 50% of the drug from the plasma (in this case, from 10 mg/100 ml to 5 mg/100 ml). By a further 2 hours, 50% of the remaining drug (5 mg/100 ml) is removed (down to 2.5 mg/100 ml). By another 2 hours again, 50% of the remaining drug (2.5 mg/100 ml) is removed (down to 1.25 mg/100 ml), and so on.

the drug not immediately available for use. Some drugs cross the blood–brain barrier and affect the neurons directly, but others are prevented from crossing the barrier. Some may only cross in **precursor** form (i.e. an earlier stage in the synthesis pathway of a chemical), and will need conversion to the final form in the neuron.

Many drugs require metabolism, usually by the liver, before excretion. The liver's action produces **metabolites**, i.e. metabolic products of the drug. Some metabolites have biological activity in the body, whilst others do not. Most drugs are excreted through the kidneys in urine, and the rate of liver metabolism and renal excretion are two important factors that influence the **half-life** of the drug (Figure 6.2). The half-life is the time it takes for the body to clear half the current dose in the blood into the urine. For example, if the dose in the blood is 60 mg (milligrams), and the half-life is one hour, then in the first hour the body would clear 30 mg; in the second hour it would clear 15 mg of the 30 mg present at the start at that hour; in the third hour it would clear 7.5 mg, and so on: half of the *current* dose is cleared each hour.

The giving of drugs to a patient presumes that the patient has an efficient liver and kidneys, and is therefore able to handle and excrete the drug. This is the case for most psychiatric patients, but the mental health nurse must also be mindful of the occasional patient who is physically unable to metabolise or excrete the drug. In this situation the patient is at risk of rapid toxicity by the presence of a drug that cannot be eliminated. Alcoholic patients are particularly at risk, since their liver is likely already to be under considerable stress from the alcohol and they may be suffering from some degree of reduced liver function. In such a patient, additional drugs may precipitate total liver failure.

Pharmacogenetics

Pharmacogenetics is the name given to the study of the effects genes have on the way the body handles drugs or the way drugs handle the body (Wolf *et al.* 2000). It has been recognised for a long time that different individuals respond to the same drug in different ways. Only more recently has the role of genes been seen as important in this different response to drugs. This means that patients with different genetic backgrounds may be given different drugs for the same condition, and that genetic testing may be required to provide more accurate drug treatment. Nurses should be aware that this is one important reason why one patient responds well to a drug while another does not.

Drug administration

Drugs are given by the **intramuscular route** for several reasons:

- For rapid absorption over just a few minutes, when speed of drug action is important, such as in a psychiatric emergency. Intravenous (IV) administration is the only route faster than intramuscular, but for IV administration accuracy is required to find a vein, and this is likely to be impossible (and undesirable) in most psychiatric emergencies. Intravenous injections of anticonvulsant drugs may, however, be the preferred option in some instances for the control of epileptic fits.
- Efficiency in administration, especially when oral drugs may be difficult to give, may be spat out by the patient, or may simply not be swallowed (known as poor **patient compliance**) (Coffey 1999).
- When a large dose is required, since the larger muscles can accommodate up to 2 millilitres (ml) of fluid.
- When drugs cannot be given by mouth because of gastric acidity or digestive enzymes that alter or destroy the drug.

Intramuscular injections are absorbed from the muscle tissue into the general (systemic) blood circulation. Water-based drugs are absorbed faster than oil-based drugs. Binding a drug to oil slows its absorption, which is useful if the drug has to be released from the muscle over a long period, thus increasing the duration of drug activity. Such injected drugs are called **depots**. One depot injection can release the drug into the blood circulation over a number of days rather than minutes, ensuring that the medication is delivered without the need for repeated daily oral doses. Absorption of a drug from the muscle is dependent on the blood supply to that muscle. In cases where the blood supply is poor, such as in shock or profound **hypotension** (low blood pressure), absorption is greatly slowed down, and may even stop. This is not usually a problem for the majority of patients.

Intradermal (or **subcutaneous**) injections are given into the dermis of the skin. This route is useful for the administration of small volumes of a drug, particularly where a slightly longer period of absorption is required than is given by the intramuscular route (e.g. in the case of insulin). Intradermal drugs are absorbed slowly into the dermal capillaries and on into the systemic veins.

Oral administration is used whenever possible for the convenience of both the patient (where patient compliance is not a problem) and the staff. It is the preferred method for most drugs that can be tolerated by the digestive system because it is noninvasive. Even where some oral drugs may be affected by the gastric acidity, **enteric coated** oral medication helps to prevent breakdown in the acidic stomach; the drug is not released until it arrives in the alkaline areas of the bowel. Some drugs (e.g. tetracycline) bind to alkaline substances and therefore should not be given with milk. Binding with milk will delay or prevent absorption from the small bowel. Giving drugs immediately after food often promotes absorption, since this is the time when the bowel is active and drugs are driven past the stomach into the bowel more quickly.

Per rectum (**PR**) and **inhaled** drugs are not used regularly in psychiatry (unless the patient also has another condition, such as asthma). Rectal drugs are absorbed relatively slowly and offer no real advantage over oral administration. Inhaled drugs are only suitable for the treatment of respiratory problems, since their main action is on the lungs, with less drug being absorbed into the systemic circulation than was first administered, giving a poor unreliable systemic activity.

Drug names

Often, drugs have three names (NPF/BNF 1999). An example is followed through here for one particular drug.

1 **Chemical name**, mostly based on the chemical structure and not used in clinical practice. (E.g. 7-chloro-1,3-dihydro-1-methyl-5-phenyl-2H-1, 4-benzodiazepin-2-one.)
2 **Official**, **approved** or **generic** name, most often used in clinical practice because this name does not identify any specific manufacturer. (E.g. diazepam.)
3 **Proprietary**, or **trade** name, given by individual manufacturers to their own products and not often used on drug prescriptions because the same drug may be produced more cheaply by another company under a different name. (E.g. Valium.)

Drug abuse

The reward pathways of the brain

One of the major quests in brain research over the past ten years or so has been to try to identify the neurological areas involved in euphoria and pleasure. This endeavour has met with some success and has resulted in the identification of some areas of the brain involved in drug addiction. As with many other functions of the brain, the so-called **reward centres** are not one or two isolated areas but rather appear to be several centres linked by reward pathways involving mostly dopamine as the neurotransmitter.

See page 19, Table 1.2

Important areas stand out as reward centres, in particular the **medial forebrain bundle,** which links the **ventral tegmental area** of the midbrain with the **nucleus accumbens** (Figure 6.3). This pathway forms part of a larger system called the **mesotelencephalic dopamine system,** a system that runs from the mesencephalon (the midbrain) to the telencephalon

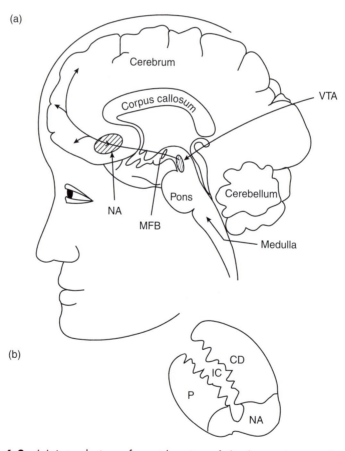

FIGURE 6.3 (a) Lateral view of a mid-section of the brain showing the medial forebrain bundle (MFB) extending from the ventral tegmental area (VTA) to the nucleus accumbens (NA). (b) The nucleus accumbens in association with the caudate nucleus (CN), internal capsule (IC) and the putamen (P).

(the end brain, or cerebrum) (Figure 6.3). The nuclei in the brain stem, from which the neurons of the mesotelencephalic system arise, are the ventral tegmental area and the substantia nigra. Apart from the nucleus accumbens, the system serves other nuclei of the telencephalon, notably the **septum** and the **prefrontal cortex** and two other important areas of the brain, the **limbic cortex** and **amygdala** (see Chapter 1). This dopamine pathway is strongly implicated in many self-administered stimulatory drug effects including those of the opiates and amphetamines. The ventral tegmental area is involved in behavioural arousal, and activation of this centre causes dopamine to be released from the synapses of the medial forebrain bundle. This dopamine binds to receptors at the nucleus accumbens, causing further activity. One such receptor, the **A1 receptor** (a variation of dopamine 2 receptor), if present, increases the risk of addiction, especially to alcohol. Like all receptors, its presence or absence depends on inheritance: the gene that codes for the A1 receptor can be passed between generations of the same family, or may be absent entirely from a family. Alcoholic fathers who have the gene can pass it to their children, who may therefore develop a higher risk of alcoholism.

Other brain areas involved in reward mechanisms, and therefore reinforcing pleasure-seeking activity, are the septum (a site of sexual pleasure, optimism, euphoria and happiness), the temporal lobes of the cerebrum and parts of the hypothalamus (Figure 6.4). The septum as well as the nucleus

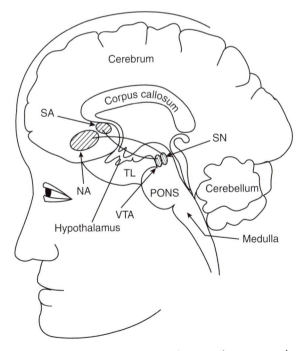

Figure 6.4 Same view as in Figure 6.3a showing the main pathways from the substantia nigra (SN) to the nucleus accumbens (NA), and from the ventral tegmental area (VTA) to the septal area (SA). TL is the temporal lobe.

accumbens also receives input from the ventral tegmental area via the medial forebrain bundle. This bundle also carries connections linking the substantia nigra (in the midbrain) with the nucleus accumbens (Figure 6.4). All of these connections are dopaminergic and stimulation of either the ventral tegmental area or parts of the substantia nigra causes an increase in dopamine levels in the nucleus accumbens during a sensation of euphoria or pleasure. It should not be a surprise, therefore, to find that many stimulant and addictive drugs are those that cause high dopamine levels to occur in the brain and in the nucleus accumbens in particular.

See page 128

Drug addiction has become the subject of increasing genetic research, especially alcoholism. Interest grew in this area mainly because of the individual variations shown by people in response to drugs, a phenomenon which is most likely to have a genetic basis. More information will become available as work continues in this new area of research.

Drug interactions

Two or more drugs inside the body can interact in ways which have a significant effect on one or both drugs involved. This effect may be beneficial to the patient, but in most cases it will be harmful.

See page 110

Pharmacokinetic interactions occur during the process of moving drugs around the body from absorption to excretion (see pharmacokinetics). The most common interactions of this sort take place during **biotransformation**, when drugs are converted to an excretable form, the metabolite, usually in the liver. Interactions between drugs can either increase (less commonly) or decrease (more commonly) the activity of the liver enzymes that carry out biotransformation, and therefore affect the bioavailabilty and half-life of either or both drugs involved. Other pharmacokinetic inter-actions involve drugs competing for protein binding in the blood or for transport mechanisms across membranes and barriers such as the blood–brain barrier.

See page 111
See page 110

See page 46

See page 108

Pharmacodynamic interactions occur at cellular level where one drug interferes with the mechanism by which another drug acts. This happens either at the cell surface receptors or inside the cell.

Drug interactions are important to the nurse who needs to be alert to the possibility of the patient obtaining illegal drugs whilst taking prescribed medication. The sections that follow provide a brief guide to the most important and best understood drug interactions.

The opiate drugs

These drugs are derived from **opium**, a resin obtained from the opium poppy. The best-known examples of the opiate derivatives are **morphine**, **heroin**, **pethidine** and **methadone**. They are all potentially addictive and dangerous; morphine and heroin together killed 754 people in the United Kingdom in 1999.

See page 56

Opiates (the word refers to the drugs) act on specific opioid receptors (opioid = 'like opium', the word refers to the endogenous neurotransmitters), which occur mostly in the upper parts of the spinal cord and the brain stem. These receptors are called **mu** (μ), **delta** (δ) and **kappa** (κ) (see subtypes of opioid receptors). Opioid receptors are metabotropic, involving the activation of the secondary messenger cAMP via a G-protein coupling mechanism. Opiate drugs cause a number of different effects on both the body and the mind, including analgesia, euphoria, sedatory and depressant effects. The effect of most importance is the euphoria and the feeling of well-being these drugs induce, as this is the reason people take them. The exact mechanism by which this effect is achieved is not fully known, but it appears to be mediated through binding, primarily to the mu receptor. At the same time, activity on this receptor causes the classic analgesic effects and reinforces drug-seeking behaviour. It also causes release of dopamine into the nucleus accumbens, a common effect of many drugs of addiction. Dopaminergic neurons of the medial forebrain bundle are inhibited by a GABA-mediated system in the ventral tegmental area. Opiate drugs reduce this inhibition, allowing dopamine to be released in the nucleus accumbens (Figure 6.5). Morphine binds mostly to the mu receptor and least of all to the delta receptor, whilst pethidine also has its greatest activity on the mu receptor. Heroin (diamorphine) is made from morphine but is more lipid-soluble and more potent than its parent molecule. Long-term use of

See page 56

See page 41

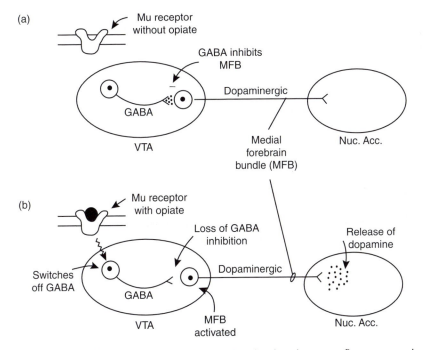

FIGURE 6.5 (a) The mu receptor without opiate binding has no influence over the GABA neurons of the ventral tegmental area (VTA). These neurons therefore inhibit the dopaminergic neurons of the medial forebrain bundle (MFB), which pass from the VTA to the nucleus accumbens (Nuc. Acc.). (b) Opiates binding to mu receptors switch off the GABA neurons, thus removing the GABA inhibition, and the MFB becomes activated, causing release of dopamine in the nucleus accumbens.

morphine and heroin causes damage to the immune system, making addicts more susceptible to infections.

Opiate addiction, as with other drugs, leads to two problems encountered by the addict. One is **withdrawal**, a set of unpleasant symptoms that occurs within hours of abstinence from the drug and can last up to three or more days. Symptoms include hot and cold flushes, loss of appetite, muscle cramps, tremor, nausea, vomiting and insomnia. Physical changes include increased heart rate and blood pressure and raised respiration rate and body temperature. While drugs are sought and taken initially for their euphoric effect (positive symptoms), drug-seeking behaviour is reinforced by the need to avoid the unpleasant effects of withdrawal (negative symptoms). This change from *nondependent* drug seeking for pleasure to *dependent* drug seeking for prevention of withdrawal could be the result of a shift in the activation of different parts of the brain. While the neurological basis of euphoria appears to be located primarily within the mesotelencephalic dopamine

See page 114

system, the neurological basis of withdrawal appears to be the result of activity of another pathway, the 'extended amygdala'. This consists of the **amygdala central medial nucleus**, part of the **stria terminalis**, part of the nucleus accumbens and the **sublenticular substantia innominata** (Figure 6.6). This system has connections with other parts of the brain through inputs (afferents) and outputs (efferents), as shown in Figure 6.6. Studies of the neurochemistry during withdrawal have indicated reduced levels of both dopamine and serotonin in the brain, i.e. *down regulation* of these systems, and increased levels (*up regulation*) of **corticotropin-releasing factor** (**CRF**) (Koob 2000). CRF is probably best known as the local hormone from the hypothalamus that enters the pituitary gland and controls the release of one of the anterior pituitary hormones called **adrenocorticotropic hormone** (**ACTH**). It is also, however, a neurotransmitter of the limbic system and is involved in emotions and stress (see Chapter 6), and in withdrawal from drugs (Carlson 2001). The mechanism involving CRF in drug craving during withdrawal is not fully known, but part of the withdrawal effect appears to involve the activation of CRF systems within the central medial nucleus of the amygdala, part of the 'extended amygdala' circuit (Koob 2000).

The second problem for the addict is that of **tolerance**, the state in which over time increasing doses of the drug become necessary to achieve anything like the original feelings of euphoria. It appears that the opioid receptors become less sensitive to the drug, a process of *down regulation* of sensitivity, although the receptor numbers remain constant. This may be due in part to the action of a protein called **cyclic AMP-responsive element-binding protein** (**CREB**). When opiates bind to the mu receptor, cAMP is produced, and this passes to the nucleus and interacts with CREB (Figure 6.7). The role of CREB is one of gene regulation, and the way in which the binding of cAMP influences this role is little understood. CREB is a major link in the chain from receptor to gene and evidence suggests it may be involved in opiate tolerance and the effects of drug withdrawal (Maldonado *et al.* 1996; Carlson 2001). Other proteins are undoubtedly important in drug addiction. A gene has recently been discovered that codes for a protein

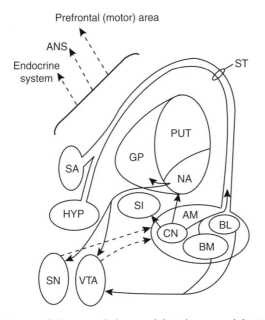

FIGURE 6.6 Pathways of the extended amygdala. The amygdala (AM) main nuclei are the central nucleus (CN), the basolateral nucleus (BL) and the basomedial nucleus (BM). Part of the stria terminalis (ST), which links the amygdala with the septal area (SA) and the hypothalamus (HYP), is involved, along with the sublenticular substantia innominata (SI), the nucleus accumbens (NA), the substantia nigra (SN), the ventral tegmental area (VTA) and the globus pallidus (GP). This system influences the prefrontal motor area (motor planning), the autonomic nervous system (ANS) and the endocrine system, the last two through the hypothalamus. PUT is the putamen.

involved in euphoria. This protein is a vital component in the pathway that leads from the brain's release of beta-endorphins to the sensation of euphoria or pleasure that these endorphins produce. Blocking the gene (dubbed the *pleasure gene*), reduces the amount of protein produced, causing loss of the euphoric state. It is thought that the same mechanism will probably also be effective in reducing the euphoric (and thus addictive) effects of opiate drugs like morphine and heroin. In the future, drugs designed to block the production of the protein may help heroin addicts to withdraw from their addiction more easily, with fewer or less intense side-effects. The analgesic qualities of these drugs do not appear be affected when this gene is blocked.

Some important *drug interactions* involving opiates with other drugs occur and are shown in Tables 6.1 and 6.2.

An important drug used as a treatment of abuse of the so-called 'hard' drugs (usually heroin and pethidine) is **methadone**. Although methadone itself is addictive and harmful, it is considered to cause fewer problems than the 'hard' drugs and for this reason has been used as a substitute for them for many years. It is hoped that by replacing heroin and pethidine with methadone not only will the need for the 'hard' drug be removed, but at the same time the effects of its withdrawal will be reduced. However, the potential

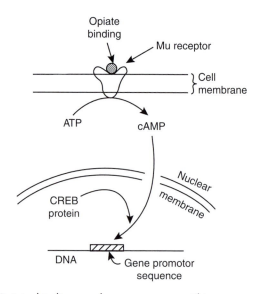

FIGURE 6.7 Opiate binding to the mu receptor. This creates cyclic adenosine monophosphate (cAMP) from adenosine triphosphate (ATP) inside the cell. cAMP influences gene expression inside the chromosomes of the nucleus by binding with CREB (cyclic AMP-responsive element-binding) protein.

TABLE 6.1 Drug interactions with opiates

Other drug	Opiate drug interaction and notes
Chlorpromazine	May react with heroin, giving uncontrolled limb jerks
Clozapine (antipsychotic)	May react with heroin, causing drowsiness
Fluoxetine (antidepressant)	May react with heroin, causing fits
MAOI (antidepressant)	Reacts with pethidine, potentially fatal
Barbiturates	Increases the metabolism of all opiate drugs

See page 196

dangers of methadone are demonstrated by the 298 deaths it caused in the United Kingdom in 1999.

Because of methadone's place in therapy, a separate drug interaction table for methadone is given in Table 6.2. Anti-HIV drugs are included in Table 6.2 because of the increased risks of drug-abusing patients being HIV positive.

Cocaine, amphetamines and other dopamine-enhancing drugs

Cocaine is produced from the leaf of the coca bush and has been used for many years as a local anaesthetic. When injected intravenously or inhaled (e.g. as *crack cocaine*, a very potent form), cocaine will reach the brain quickly,

TABLE 6.2 Drug interactions with methadone

Other drug	Methadone interaction and notes	
Phenobarbitone	Phenobarbitone blocks the action of methadone causing opioid withdrawal symptoms	
Diazepam, and other benzodiazepine drugs	Inhibits methadone metabolism causing increased methadone blood levels	*See page 155*
Tricyclic antidepressants	Methadone blocks the metabolism of the antidepressant, increasing the blood level of the antidepressant	*See page 194*
Hypnotics (e.g. zopiclone and chlormethiazole)	Increased sedative effect with methadone	
SSRI antidepressants	Increased levels of methadone in the blood	*See page 195*
Disulfiram (anti-alcohol drug)	Some methadone products contain alcohol; a reaction with these products can be alarming and unpleasant	*See page 129*
Other opiate drugs	Increased sedation and respiratory depression	
Naloxone (opiate antagonist)	Blocks methadone action causing withdrawal	
Alcohol	Increase sedation and respiratory depression; increased liver toxicity	*See page 127*
Nevirapine, zidovudine and ritonavir (anti-HIV drugs)	Nevirapine causes increased methadone metabolism, i.e. lower blood methadone levels. Methadone raises blood level of zidovudine. Ritonavir may raise blood methadone levels by blocking methadone metabolism	

causing a sense of well-being, euphoria, alertness and increased energy; the person taking it becomes extraverted, restless and talkative. It also causes a reduction in food intake. Cocaine is extremely addictive, partly owing to its rapid transportation to the brain and fast onset of effects, and at high dosages the user becomes unable to sleep and has tremors, nausea and psychotic outbursts (hallucinations, delusions, mood disturbance and bizarre behaviour; the so-called *cocaine psychosis*). Fits and unconsciousness may follow, with a corresponding risk of death.

Cocaine blocks the re-uptake of monoamines, especially dopamine and noradrenaline, into the presynaptic bulb by inhibiting the pumps (or transporters) in the presynaptic membrane (Figure 6.8). These neurotransmitters then accumulate in the cleft, exerting a greater than normal effect on the receptors. Areas of the brain affected include the basal ganglia (putamen and caudate nucleus), the amygdala and the cerebral cortex.

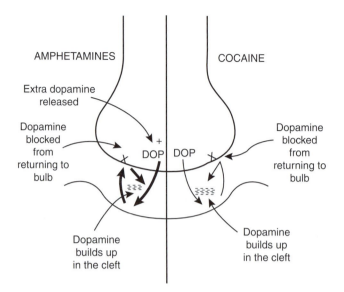

FIGURE 6.8 The action of amphetamines (left) and cocaine (right) at the dopaminergic synapse. Dopamine (DOP) is blocked from reabsorption back into the presynaptic bulb by both drugs, thus increasing the quantity of dopamine within the synaptic cleft. In addition, amphetamines increase the quantity of dopamine released from the bulb.

However, the nucleus accumbens is particularly affected, with long-term changes in this area occurring following exposure to the drug. These changes involve an increase in the density of dopamine receptors, notably D_3, and can cause a rapid return to psychotic symptoms on re-exposure to the drug even after quite some time without it.

A single dose of cocaine has been shown to cause major changes in the brain resulting in memory loss and addiction, due to its prolonged neuroleptic action of about a week's duration (Ungless *et al.* 2001). This action interferes with the normal process of memory and renders the brain vulnerable to successive doses, leading to rapid addiction. Users 'remember' the euphoria and this reinforces further drug abuse. Cocaine is also responsible for a quarter of the nonfatal heart attacks found in those younger than 45 years of age. The drug causes cardiac spasms and induces the immune system to destroy cardiac muscle cells. Deaths from cocaine use in the United Kingdom increased sevenfold in the six years from 1993, i.e. 12 deaths in 1993 compared to 87 deaths in 1999.

One possible way of treating cocaine addiction in the future may be with a cocaine vaccine. The vaccine stimulates production of antibodies which lock onto cocaine, forming a complex which is too large to cross the blood–brain barrier and thus preventing cocaine from entering the brain.

Some important *drug interactions* involving cocaine with other drugs occur and are shown in Table 6.3.

Amphetamines act in a way similar to cocaine, i.e. they increase dopamine (and noradrenaline) levels within the synapses by blocking their re-uptake, but they also have the additional effect of increasing dopamine release from

TABLE 6.3 Drug interactions with cocaine

Other drug	Interaction with cocaine
Alcohol	Increased euphoric effect. Increased heart rate and blood cortisol levels
Heroin	Increased euphoria
Lithium	Decreases the effect of the cocaine
MAOI antidepressant	High temperature, muscle rigidity and tremor, coma
Antipsychotics	Increase in the positive (psychotic) symptoms of cocaine (see *cocaine psychosis*)
Calcium channel blockers (anti-epileptic)	Reduce the cardiac effects of cocaine, but may increase the risk of fits
Beta-adrenergic blockers (cardiac drugs)	Increased risk of cocaine-induced constriction of the coronary artery (i.e. risk of myocardial ischaemia)

the presynaptic bulb (Figure 6.8). Amphetamines were responsible for 79 deaths in the United Kingdom during the year 1999.

Ecstasy (**3,4-methylenedioxymethamphetamine**, or **MDMA**) is one of a group of related amphetamine-associated drugs. MDMA is converted in the body to the active metabolite **4-hydroxy-3-methoxymethamphetamine** (**HMMA**). Ecstasy increases the release of serotonin into the synapses of the serotonergic diffuse modulatory system by causing the transporters that normally facilitate serotonin re-uptake to reverse the flow into the synapse. The larger amounts of serotonin released in this way increase the 'high' that users experience (Concar 2002). HMMA is associated with an increased release of the pituitary hormone **ADH** (**antidiuretic hormone**, or **vasopressin**) (Figure 6.9). This hormone reabsorbs water back into the blood from the kidney, preventing its loss in the urine. The extra water in the blood dilutes the plasma electrolytes and this shift in plasma salts level affects neurons, which are sensitive to electrolyte levels in their extracellular fluid. The brain becomes swollen with water, and drinking more water accelerates the harmful effects. Women are particularly vulnerable to this effect since the female hormone estrogen speeds up the process. High levels of circulating estrogen occur just prior to ovulation, about midway through the ovarian cycle; women at this point may already be suffering some disturbance in cerebral sodium levels, putting them more at risk from the effects of Ecstasy. The brain reacts to the MDMA-induced excess water with convulsions and coma, often leading to death within a few hours or days. There were five deaths from MDMA in the United Kingdom in 1998, and there have been about 100 since then, i.e. about a dozen deaths per year. However, there was a worrying sharp increase in deaths reported for 2001 despite the media coverage highlighting the dangers. The deaths occur mostly in the under-30 age range; the risks vary between individuals because of sexual and genetic differences.

See page 184

See page 112

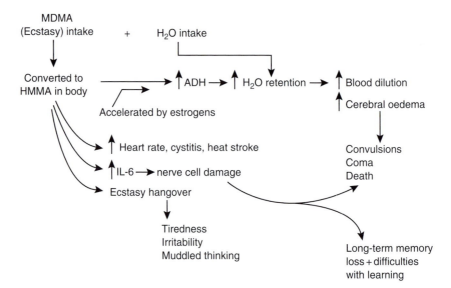

FIGURE 6.9 Ecstasy intake and the events that follow. ADH = antidiuretic hormone, H_2O = water, IL-6 = interleukin-6.

In the majority of Ecstasy takers who survive, other physical changes take place including increased heart rate, cystitis and heavy periods in women, heatstroke (Blows 1998; Concar 2002) and possible **cerebral infarcts** if blood capillaries become blocked in the brain. MDMA also interferes with the immune system by raising the levels of a chemical called **interleukin-6 (IL-6)**, which at the new higher levels damages nerve cells, particularly the serotonergic neurons. This puts the user at higher risk of infections. In the brain, MDMA initially gives a sense of euphoria, but it seriously affects the serotonin pathways, causing damage to areas of the cerebral cortex and hippocampus. This damage can occur quickly, within four days of Ecstasy use, and the damage is permanent, causing memory losses and difficulties with learning for years. Long-term widespread use of the drug could result in a whole generation of people with memory problems who will have difficulty in carrying out simple mental tasks. As many as 500 000 Ecstasy users in the United Kingdom and 20 million people worldwide could be affected in this way. After use, Ecstasy can cause a hangover effect similar to that induced by alcohol (the **Ecstasy hangover**) with tiredness, irritability and muddled thinking, due to the decline in the levels of serotonin.

Some important *drug interactions* involving amphetamines with other drugs occur and are shown in Table 6.4.

Cannabinoids

Marihuana comes from the dried leaves of the Indian hemp plant called **Cannabis sativa**. The active ingredients consist of more than 80 **cannabinoids**, many of which are probably psychoactive. The most potent of these is **delta-9-tetrahydrocannabinol (delta-9-THC** or **Δ⁹-THC)**. After

TABLE 6.4 Drug interactions with amphetamines

Other drug	Interaction with amphetamines
MAOI antidepressants	Dangerous interaction: risk of hypertensive crisis due to raised sympathetic nervous system activity (i.e. sympathomimetic); plus nausea, cardiac arrhythmias and chest pain
Opiates	Increased analgesic effect of the opiate
Chlorpromazine (antipsychotic)	Both drugs are reduced in their efficiency causing an increase in psychotic symptoms
Lithium	Reduces the amphetamine euphoria

absorption, this substance binds to cannabinoid receptors in several parts of the brain, notably the basal ganglia, the hippocampus, the cerebellum and the frontal lobe of the cerebrum. The effects of taking cannabinoids in sufficient dosage are alterations in cognition, euphoria and other mood and emotional changes. A sense of unreality with sensory distortion, slurred speech, analgesia (without respiratory depression), sedation and suppression of the immune system have all been reported. The reason for taking the drug – that is, the euphoric effect produced – is probably due to its ability to raise dopamine levels within the nucleus accumbens. The mood changes and loss of short-term memory linked to the use of marihuana are probably due to hippocampal involvement. The hippocampus has particularly high numbers of cannabinoid receptors and therefore the drug may act especially here, resulting not only in impairment of short-term memory but also in disruption of release of cortisol, a hormone involved in mood regulation. An important function of the hippocampus is regulation of some hormones, including cortisol.

Cannabinoid receptors occur in at least two known subtypes, **CB$_1$** and **CB$_2$**. CB$_1$ is the major cannabinoid receptor subtype of the central nervous system (CNS), with CB$_2$ in the brain limited to possibly only the cerebellum (it occurs more in other organs). Apart from the hippocampal effects, the drugs acting on CB$_1$ receptors in the basal ganglia can cause loss of control of voluntary movements, the addition of involuntary movements and **akinesia** (a loss of initiating a movement). CB$_1$ receptors are especially predominant in the globus pallidus, the substantia nigra (pars reticulata) and the caudate and putamen. In the limbic system, there are significant levels of CB$_1$ receptors in the amygdala, an area central to the control of emotional responses, and in the hypothalamus, the control centre of body temperature. The cerebellum has some areas with dense levels of CB$_1$ receptors, enough to cause disturbance to motor function and balance given sufficient dosage of the drug. Levels of CB$_1$ receptors in the brain stem and spinal cord are lower than in these previously mentioned areas.

Some evidence has emerged that cannabinoids have effects similar to those of the so-called 'hard' drugs (heroin in particular), not only causing

See page 116

the dopamine release in the nucleus accumbens noted above but also causing high levels of CRF release during withdrawal (see opiates) (Concar 1997). This has led to further speculation and controversy about whether the use of cannabis can lead to addiction to hard drugs like heroin. The risk of addiction to cannabis itself has always been considered to be low, usually because it is only used occasionally and because users give up smoking the drug in their thirties or forties. Recently, however, there have been indications that cannabis is as potentially addictive as heroin or morphine (Concar 1997).

The presence of natural receptors for cannabinoids suggests that the nervous system must produce its own endogenous cannabinoid substance and the discovery of **anandamide**, an unsaturated fatty acid, confirmed this. Anandamide, produced by neurons of the cortex and parts of the basal ganglia, binds to CB_1 receptors, producing analgesia, reduced levels of movement and hypothermia (a hypothalamic effect). Its duration of action is short owing to rapid breakdown to arachidonic acid in neurons and astrocytes.

Some medical uses of cannabinoids are becoming better recognised. Their anti-emetic quality has been used for some time in the drug **nabilone** to prevent nausea and sickness in patients having chemotherapy in cancer treatment. Some cannabinoids have been shown to reduce fits, dilate the bronchus in asthma and improve the eye disease glaucoma. Now the beneficial analgesic qualities of cannabinoids may become available to multiple sclerosis sufferers if the legal issues surrounding marihuana can be resolved.

Some important *drug interactions* involving cannabinoids with other drugs occur and are shown in Table 6.5.

TABLE 6.5 Drug interactions with cannabinoids

Other drugs	Interactions with cannabinoids
Fluoxetine (SSRI antidepressant)	Increased energy and sexuality
Tricyclic antidepressant	Tachycardia and restlessness, orthostatic hypotension, sedation and unstable body temperature
Lithium	Increased blood levels of lithium, which in turn may reduce the effect of the cannabinoid
Opiates	Increased heart rate and respiratory depression
Cocaine	Raised blood levels of cocaine, causing increased cocaine activity
Amphetamines	Increased and sustained heart rate
Propranolol (cardiac drug)	Blocks the increased heart rate and blood pressure associated with cannabinoids

Alcohol

Alcohol (ethyl alcohol or ethanol) is a psychoactive drug with a small molecular size and therefore reaches all parts of the body quickly after absorption. In a low dose it acts as a *mild stimulant*, giving a feeling of well-being, and this is the reason for the *social* drinking of alcohol. However, if too much alcohol is taken it becomes a *depressant*, shutting down many areas of brain activity. Such depressive effects include cognitive impairment (i.e. distorted thinking), slowed reaction times (one good reason for not driving after drinking), verbal impairment (slurring of speech) and motor impairment (inability to stand up or walk a straight line). Very high doses (i.e. a blood level greater than 0.5% or 5 mg/dl) can cause unconsciousness and a risk of death from respiratory suppression. One in every eight young male deaths in the United Kingdom each year is caused by alcohol, either directly or indirectly, through drink-related accidents and violence. This constitutes 12.8% of British men aged 15–29 years, and 8.3% of British women of equivalent age.

Alcohol also has a dilatory effect on peripheral blood vessels, taking blood from the core towards the skin (the red nose effect). Blood flushing the skin makes the skin *feel* warmer, but actually this blood moves more heat from the body's core and that actually cools down the body temperature. It seems at odds with the way they *feel* to say that alcohol makes the person colder. However, in this situation, the brandy barrel carried by the rescue dog is not the best thing a very cold person needs when trapped in snow. Alcohol abuse over time causes both tolerance (the individual can consume more and more without undue effect) and dependence (the person needs alcohol in order to get through the day). Quick withdrawal from a long-term drinking habit causes nausea, vomiting, headache and tremors, as well as **delirium tremens** (known as the **DTs**), a collection of symptoms including agitation, confusion, tachycardia, hallucinations and delusions. The person can also become **hyperthermic** (raised body temperature) because alcohol is no longer causing heat loss.

Korsakoff syndrome is a chronic state of **amnesia** (memory loss) and **Wernicke's encephalopathy** is a state of intellectual impairment; these often occur together in a patient with long-term alcohol abuse. Both syndromes are thought to be due to a combination of factors, notably the deficiency of the vitamin called **thiamin** (vitamin B_1), alcohol neurotoxicity and hepatic dysfunction (Roberts *et al.* 1993). Distinguishing one syndrome from the other in chronic alcoholic patients is not always easy. Many alcoholics lack nutrients as they tend not to eat properly, and chronic alcohol abuse results in gastric damage which impedes the absorption of vitamins, particularly thiamin. These factors lead to a degeneration of the brain stem (periaquaductal grey), the hypothalamus (mammillary bodies) and the thalamus (dorsomedial nucleus). Korsakoff syndrome is characterised by a loss of short-term memory, inability to learn new skills, disorientation and confabulation to fill in missing gaps in knowledge. This is often considered to be a late phase of Wernicke's encephalopathy. The features of Wernicke's encephalopathy are rapid eye movements with double vision (**diplopia**), reduced muscle coordination and a decline in mental ability that may be of any degree from mild to severe. Some recovery may be possible provided the damage is not severe and the patient abstains from alcohol for at least six months.

See page 52

Alcohol acts at the **GABA$_A$** receptor site and promotes GABA to open the chloride channels (Figure 3.17). This increases the inhibitory effect of the GABA synapses and shuts down brain activity by reducing the firing rate of neurons. People have varying responses to alcohol and not every drinker is equally at risk of becoming alcoholic. Two basic types of drinkers have been identified: the steady drinker and the binger. Steady drinking has a strong genetic basis, a case of 'like father like son'. If the father has a history of alcohol abuse, the son has a seven times greater risk of abusing alcohol than the son of a non-drinker. The daughters of drinking fathers do not show the same degree of slide into alcoholism as the sons, but they do tend to complain more about physical symptoms for which pathology cannot be found; a condition known as **somatisation disorder**. No data appear to be available for the offspring of alcoholic mothers. Steady drinking starts early in life and is associated with many kinds of antisocial behaviour, such as fighting, impulsive actions and lack of remorse. Bingeing alcohol abuse has a greater environmental than genetic cause. The father-to-child hereditary pattern is only activated in an environment where the child is exposed to bouts of heavy drinking. Bingers start drinking later in life and can be of either sex. They show increased emotional states and anxiety, become rigid in their outlook, fearful of any changes, cautious and sensitive to social cues.

See page 115

See page 45

See page 115

The genetic basis of alcoholism has become the subject of greater interest with the sequencing of the human genome. It became particularly important with the discovery of the *A1* allele on chromosome 11. This particular allele is a variation of the gene that codes for the dopamine receptor known as D$_2$, and its presence increases the risk of alcohol abuse. Of all severe alcoholics, 56.3% have the *A1* allele compared with only 25.7% of a control population. Given that dopamine is involved in the reward pathways of the brain, it may be that the *A1* allele is also linked to increased risk of abuse of other drugs.

Some important *drug interactions* involving alcohol with other drugs occur and are shown in Table 6.6. Nurses need to be aware of these interactions because of the common social nature of alcohol consumption, but particularly in the known alcoholic patient who may be taking other medication.

Nicotine

The two biggest health problems of this century are **human immuno-deficiency virus** (**HIV**, the causative agent of **acquired immunodeficiency syndrome**, or **AIDS**) and **tobacco smoking**. Both problems are increasing globally. Any individual in the Western world who can avoid both HIV and tobacco has a life expectancy of 70 years at least, and often more. Both these problems are relevant to this chapter because HIV infection is a major risk to intravenous drug abusers who share contaminated needles, and

TABLE 6.6 Drug interactions with alcohol

Other drug	Interaction with alcohol
Barbiturates; warfarin; phenytoin; rifampicin	Interaction varies according to how much alcohol is consumed. Heavy drinking increases at least one liver enzyme activity, withdrawal decreases that activity
Paracetamol	Alcohol increases activity of the liver enzyme that acts on paracetamol, causing increased toxicity of paracetamol at normally nontoxic dose. Overdose of paracetamol with alcohol can cause lethal liver failure
Opiates; benzodiazepines	Alcohol adds to the depressive effect of the drugs on the brain
Tricyclic antidepressants	Unexpected reactions and behavioural changes. Lower blood levels of the tricyclic reduces clinical effects
SSRI antidepressants	No known interaction
MAOI antidepressants	Risk of hypertension, especially if tyromine is present in the alcoholic drink. Modern reversible MAOI may not be such a problem
Antipsychotics	Poor psychomotor skills and impaired nervous system function
Disulfiram (anti-alcohol)	Flushing, hypotension, nausea, increased heart rate, some reactions could be fatal
Nonsteroidal anti-inflammatory drugs	Increased risk of gastrointestinal bleeds since alcohol is a gastric irritant
Insulin	Too much alcohol causes severe and prolonged hypoglycaemia in diabetic patients, following lowering of stored liver glycogen
Antihypertensive drugs	Increased risk of postural hypotension

tobacco contains the addictive drug nicotine. Nicotine addiction is a major hazard, causing the deaths of about 300 people per day in the United Kingdom alone from smoking-related diseases, and smoking in young women in particular is increasing at alarming rates. Nicotine addiction must not be underestimated. Addiction to this drug prevents many people who want to give up smoking from doing so. Only about 20% of people attempting to stop smoking are successful two years after abstaining from cigarettes, and this applies when they are faced with serious health problems or even death. A vaccine against nicotine, now in an advanced stage of development, may be instrumental in the treatment of nicotine addiction and in prevention.

Like most addictive drugs, nicotine increases the level of dopamine in the nucleus accumbens, but also raises the activity levels of many dopaminergic neurons. Evidence is now pointing towards smoking tobacco as an important

TABLE 6.7 The effects of inhaling nicotine on non-smokers and smokers

Non-smokers	Smokers
Various combinations of nausea, vomiting, coughing, sweating, dizziness, flushing of the face, even abdominal cramps and diarrhoea	Relaxation, alertness, reduced hunger

TABLE 6.8 Drug interactions with nicotine

Other drugs	Interactions with nicotine
Benzodiazepines	Increased activity of the liver enzymes that metabolise the benzodiazepines, causing reduced efficiency of these drugs

cause of anxiety states, depression and perhaps other mental health disorders, due in part to the increased dopaminergic activity that nicotine causes in the brain (Petit-Zeman 2002). Table 6.7 demonstrates the effects of inhaling nicotine on both non-smokers and smokers. Given these differences, it becomes obvious how tolerance to nicotine changes a person's perception of the drug and how intolerable passive smoking is to the non-smoker.

Very few known *drug interactions* involving nicotine with other drugs occur (Table 6.8). Other interactions probably do occur but they remain unstudied. Smoking is a common habit, not least amongst those under treatment for mental health disorders. Combinations of prescribed drugs with nicotine may be a problem that nurses should be aware of.

The hallucinogenic drugs

One of the most potent hallucinogenic agents is **lysergic acid diethylamide** (**LSD**), which produces a dream-like state with heightened senses and a strange blending of those senses such that, for example, visual images can cause sounds or weird smells. During the early stages of LSD administration the effect is of witnessing abstract coloured geometric shapes, such as parallel stripes, hexagons and checkers. This is followed by the appearance of four specific forms: tunnels, spirals, cobwebs and honeycomb patterns (Figure 6.10). This phenomenon is akin to **hallucinations**, i.e. sensing something that is not real, and the study of these effects may give clues to the origin of psychotic hallucinations. Under the influence of LSD, neurons in the visual sensory area of the brain (area VI, Brodmann 17, in the occipital lobe) fire even when there is nothing on the retina to see (Mackenzie 2001).

See page 6

The chemical structure of LSD is very similar to that of serotonin and this means it probably works on the serotonergic pathways of the brain stem. It certainly causes less serotonin to be secreted in the raphe nucleus of the brain stem. Serotonin usually has an inhibitory function on other brain

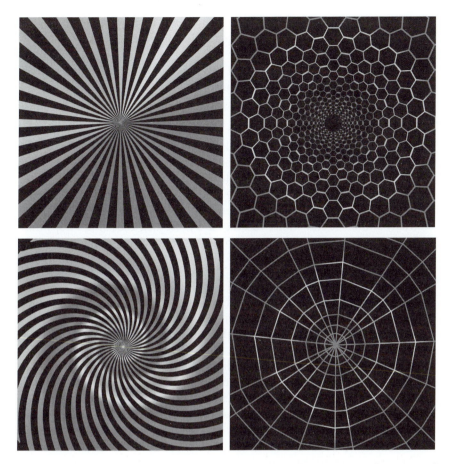

FIGURE 6.10 The patterns of hallucinations witnessed during an LSD (lysergic acid diethylamide) 'trip' consists of webs, spirals, honeycombs and tunnels in vivid multi-colours. Reproduced with permission of New Scientist (issue 2296, 23rd June 2001)

areas and the LSD-induced lower secretion removes this inhibition, so the brain become more active.

Phencyclidine (**PCP**) is another hallucinogen, causing excitement, agitation, delirium and mixed, disorganised perception. It is an NMDA receptor antagonist and causes the release of dopamine. Another less potent NMDA receptor antagonist is the anaesthetic **ketamine**, which can also cause brief dreamlike states and psychotic symptoms. The brain pathways along which these drugs act are speculative, but may lie in the prefrontal cortex of the cerebrum.

See page 49

Key points

Pharmacodynamics

- The two basic drug actions are the agonist and the antagonist. Agonist drugs bind to and activate receptors. Antagonist drugs also bind to but block receptors, preventing the binding of the natural ligand.

- Other drugs affect the level of neurotransmitter in the synapse by inhibiting the re-uptake into the bulb, or by blocking the enzyme that breaks down the neurotransmitter.
- Some drugs reduce the number of action potentials by blocking sodium or calcium channels, and thus reduce brain activity.

The reward pathways

- The medial forebrain bundle links the ventral tegmental area of the midbrain with the nucleus accumbens of the cerebral frontal lobe. This pathway forms part of the mesotelencephalic dopamine system.
- This dopamine pathway is strongly implicated in the activities of many self-administered stimulatory drugs.
- Many stimulant and addictive drugs are those that cause high dopamine levels to occur in the brain, and in the nucleus accumbens in particular.

Opiate drugs

- Opiate drugs cause analgesia, euphoria, sedatory and depressant effects.
- The mechanism that leads to euphoria and the feeling of well-being appears to be mediated through the mu (μ) receptor, which also reinforces drug-seeking behaviour.
- The change from nondependent drug seeking for pleasure to dependent drug seeking for prevention of withdrawal could be the result of a shift to the activation of the 'extended amygdala'.
- Withdrawal from drugs is associated with reduced levels of both dopamine and serotonin in the brain, and increased levels of corticotropin-releasing factor (CRF).
- Tolerance appears to result from receptors becoming less sensitive to the drug, which may involve a protein called cyclic AMP-responsive element-binding protein (CREB).

Cocaine and amphetamines

- Cocaine blocks the re-uptake of dopamine and noradrenaline into the presynaptic bulb by inhibiting dopamine pumps in the synaptic membrane.
- Amphetamines increase dopamine and noradrenaline levels within the synapses by blocking their re-uptake, plus increasing dopamine release from the presynaptic bulb.
- Ecstasy (MDMA) is converted in the body to an active metabolite (HMMA), which causes increased antidiuretic hormone (vasopressin).
- ADH increases water in the blood, and this extra water dilutes the electrolytes around the neurons. The brain becomes swollen and suffers convulsions, coma and death.

Cannabinoids

- Marihuana comes from the dried leaves of the Indian hemp plant called *Cannabis sativa*.

- The psychoactive ingredients are cannabinoids.
- The most potent is delta-9-tetrahydrocannabinol (delta-9-THC or Δ^9-THC), which binds to cannabinoid receptors in the brain, notably the basal ganglia, the hippocampus, the cerebellum and the frontal lobe of the cerebrum.
- Cannabinoids cause not only dopamine release in the nucleus accumbens but also high levels of CRF release during withdrawal.

Alcohol

- Alcohol (ethyl alcohol or ethanol) is a psychoactive drug which in low dosage acts as a mild stimulant, giving a feeling of well-being.
- In higher doses, alcohol is a depressant to many parts of the brain. Depressive effects include cognitive impairment, slowed reaction times, and verbal and motor impairment.
- Very high doses can cause unconsciousness and death.
- Rapid withdrawal from alcohol causes nausea, vomiting, headache and tremors, as well as delirium tremens (DTs), i.e. agitation, confusion, tachycardia, hallucinations and delusions.
- Korsakoff syndrome is a chronic state of amnesia with confabulation and Wernicke's encephalopathy is a state of intellectual impairment; these occur often together in a patient with long-term alcohol abuse.
- There are two basic types of drinkers: the steady drinkers and the bingers.
- Steady drinking has a strong genetic basis, starting early in life, and is associated with antisocial behaviour.
- Bingeing alcohol abuse is more environmental than genetic in origin. It starts later in life and affects both sexes.

Nicotine

- Nicotine causes major problems of addiction, and tobacco smoking causes about 300 deaths per day in the United Kingdom alone.
- Nicotine increases the level of dopamine in the nucleus accumbens.

References

Blows W. T. (1998) Crowd physiology: the 'penguin effect'. *Accident and Emergency Nursing*, **6** (3): 126–129.

Carlson N. (2001) *Physiology of Behaviour*. Allyn and Bacon, Boston.

Concar D. (1997) A dangerous pathway. *New Scientist*, 5 July: 4.

Concar D. (2002) Ecstasy on the brain. *New Scientist*, **174** (2339; 20 April): 26–33.

Coffey M. (1999) Psychosis and medication: Strategies for improving adherence. *British Journal of Nursing*, **8** (4): 225–230.

Kaplan H. I. and Sudock B. J. (1996) *Concise Textbook of Clinical Psychiatry*. Williams and Wilkins, Baltimore.

Koob G. F. (2000) Opiate tolerance and dependence. *Science and Medicine*, **7** (2): 28–37.

MacKenzie D. (2001) Secrets of an acid head. *New Scientist*, **170** (2296; 23 June): 26–30.

Maldonado R., Blendy J. A., Tzavara E., Gass P., Roques B. P., Hanoune J. and Schutz G. (1996) Reduction of morphine abstinence in mice with a mutation in the gene encoding CREB. *Science*, **273**: 657–659.

NPF/BNF (1999) *Nurse Prescriber's Formulary and British National Formulary* 1999–2001. British Medical Association and the Royal Pharmaceutical Society of Great Britain.

Petit-Zeman S. (2002) Smoke gets in your mind. *New Scientist*, **174** (2338; 13 April): 30–33.

Roberts G. W., Leigh P. N. and Weinberger D. R. (1993) *Neuropsychiatric Disorders*. Wolfe, London.

Ungless M. A., Whistler J. L., Malenka R. C. and Bonci A. (2001) Single cocaine exposure *in vivo* induces long-term potentiation in dopamine neurons. *Nature*, **411** (31 May): 583–587.

Wolf C. R., Smith G. and Smith R. L. (2000) Pharmacogenetics. *British Medical Journal*, **320**: 987–990.

Chapter 7

Anxiety, fear and emotions

- The limbic system and the biology of emotions
- The biology of stress
- The emotions of life experiences
- Anxiety disorders
- Fear, aggression and phobic states
- Eating disorders
- Key points

The limbic system and the biology of emotions

The limbic system is a series of centres collectively involved in preservation of the individual (*self-preservation*) and *preservation of the species*. It governs behaviour essential to the survival of the individual, ensuring, for example, that we seek food or respond to threats, and also promotes reproductive behaviour (see Chapter 1) to ensure survival of the species. The major components of the limbic system (Figure 7.1) are the amygdala; the mammillary bodies of the hypothalamus; the anterior and dorsal nuclei of the thalamus; several deep nuclei; the septal area; the orbitofrontal cortex of the cerebrum; several other areas of the cortex, such as the hippocampus; the parahippocampal gyrus and parts of the temporal lobe, together known as the **limbic cortex** because of their close association with the functions of the limbic system.

See page 7

The limbic centre has the following functions:

- It is the centre for the control of emotions, including fear and aggression.
- It controls reproductive behaviour.

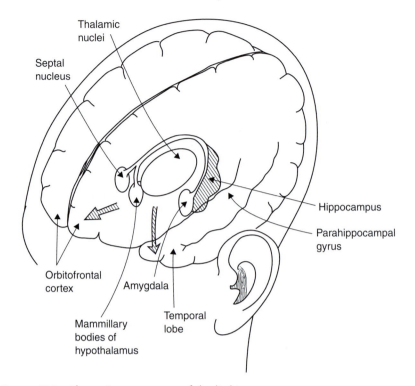

FIGURE 7.1 The main components of the limbic system.

See page 10

- It influences memory because the hippocampus stores short-term memory.
- Through the hypothalamus, it influences hormonal release and the autonomic nervous system.

See page 8

The whole system is set in a ring structure (limbic = bordering, fringeing or ringing) deep in the brain (see Chapter 1, and Figures 1.4, 1.5, and 7.1).

See page 8

The **amygdala** (Figure 7.2) is a pea-sized collection of nuclei situated within the limbic system inside the temporal lobes, below the level of the cortex. It sits at the end of the tail of the caudate nucleus (Figure 1.4). The important nuclei of the amygdala and their functions are listed below.

1 The *corticomedial* group is very small and not well defined in humans. It plays a role in inhibiting aggressive behaviour.
2 The *basolateral* group relays sensory information from the primary sensory cortex of the cerebrum (Brodmann 1, 2 and 3), the sensory association cortex (Brodmann 40) and the thalamus to the central nucleus.
3 The central nucleus receives the information from the basolateral group and has its output to the brain stem and the hypothalamus (see Figure 7.3). The output to the brain stem is to various nuclei which carry out different functions in relation to emotional reactions. The output to the hypothalamus causes physical responses by influencing hypothalamic control of both the sympathetic nervous system

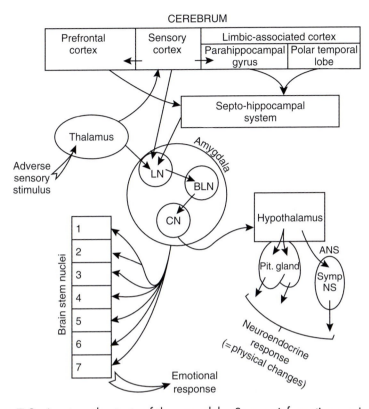

FIGURE 7.2 Inputs and outputs of the amygdala. Sensory information coming into the thalamus is passed to the sensory cortex, but also directly to the lateral nucleus (LN) of the amygdala. The sensory cortex passes the information to the prefrontal cortex to produce an action plan, which is passed to the septo-hippocampal system. Information identifying the sensory information passes through the limbic-associated cortex to the septo-hippocampal system. From here, input to the amygdala is via the lateral nucleus, to the basolateral nucleus (BLN) and on to the central nucleus (CN). The central nucleus has outputs to the brain stem nuclei (for emotional response), and the hypothalamus (for physical response).

and the pituitary hormones (collectively known as a **neuroendocrine response**).

The amygdala receives input from several sources, as listed at (2) above, with slightly delayed time intervals. The following text should be read in conjunction with Figure 7.2.

Primary amygdala input. The primary input to the amygdala is the direct automatic input of unconscious sensory stimuli from the thalamus, just as they are received from the environment. This unprocessed (or *raw*) data is the first to arrive at the amygdala and for a brief moment it is all the structure has to work on to determine the emotional response. As a result there is a rapid but not always appropriate response. The amygdala simply gives the individual the best option for survival, responding in a protective

See page 149

manner that may turn out to be unnecessary. Impulsive reactions and behaviour can be seen as *acting without thinking* or as the amygdala acting on unconscious and unconsidered, and therefore unprocessed, stimuli (note here an interesting correlation with murderers). It should not be surprising that impulsive behaviour of this kind is often seen in children, since a child's limbic system is immature. The processing and consideration of sensory stimuli requires sophisticated and complex neural systems, coupled with extensive memory stores, both of which the young brain has not had time to develop fully.

Not only has the sensory stimulus gone from the thalamus to the amygdala, but the thalamus has also passed the raw stimulus on to the primary sensory cortex of the cerebrum (if the stimulus comes from the body) or to one of the specialist sensory areas such as hearing or vision. Here the task of interpretation takes place to determine what the stimulus actually is. This involves comparing the new stimulus with memories of previous stimuli to find a match. The cerebrum adds a conscious element to the stimulus, so the individual is aware of the stimulus and can add a degree of reason to the response.

Secondary amygdala input. The secondary input to the amygdala comes from the cerebral cortex. This cerebral output also passes to the **limbic-associated cortex**, which is made up of the **parahippocampal gyrus** and the **polar temporal lobe cortex**. The limbic-associated cortex consists of those areas of the cerebral cortex which work with the limbic system in the determination of stimuli. It should not be surprising to find the cerebrum and limbic system working together on emotions, since the limbic system does not have extensive memory banks to use in the identification and evaluation of stimuli. Most of the memory banks for this are found in the sensory association areas of the cerebrum. Thus it is in the limbic association cortex that interpretations and evaluation of the stimulus are mostly made: the polar temporal lobe cortex evaluates the stimulus for potential danger to the individual. The sensory cortex also sends the stimulus to the **prefrontal cortex**, where an action plan is formulated in response to the stimulus. The prefrontal cortex is close to the main motor cortex that activates skeletal muscle, so any action plan, such as running away or fighting, can be rapidly implemented. The outputs from the prefrontal cortex and the limbic-associated cortex are passed to the **septo-hippocampal system**, consisting of the **septum** and the **hippocampus**. Here integration of the action plan with the interpretation and evaluation of danger can take place, with input from short-term memory and perhaps aggression control if needed, since these are both functions of the hippocampus.

Tertiary amygdala input. The tertiary input to the amygdala is the final output from the septo-hippocampal system. The amygdala now has all the relevant information necessary to determine an appropriate emotional response.

We can put all this together in a simple scenario. Your friend decides to play a joke on you. She hides behind the door with the intention of jumping out and surprising you. As you enter the room she does just that, springing out and making a loud noise. The *primary and secondary amygdala inputs* would occur so close together that they would appear to be simultaneous.

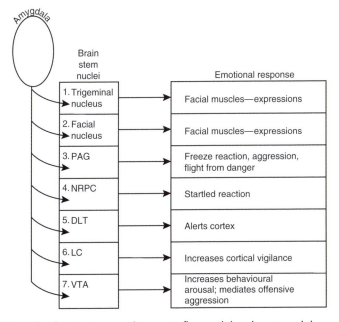

FIGURE 7.3 The brain stem nuclei are influenced by the amygdala to achieve various emotional responses, depending on which nucleus is activated. PAG = periaqueductal grey; NRPC = nucleus reticularis pontis caudalis; DLT = dorsal lateral tegmental nucleus; LC = locus coeruleus; VTA = ventral tegmental area.

You would become aware of the sudden appearance of someone jumping out at the same time as hearing a loud noise. This could be anyone or anything, a potential threat to safety. In a purely automatic defensive strategy, you are likely to attempt to move out of danger and perhaps lash out physically. This may be coupled with a scream, or some brisk language, and very rapid changes in physiology – for example, the cardiovascular system would show a dramatic rise in the pulse rate and blood pressure. But very quickly the *tertiary amygdala input*, hot on the heels of the previous two inputs, will allow some recognition of who this person is and what their intentions were.

The outputs from the amygdala (Figure 7.3) can activate:

1 Various nuclei of the **brain stem** which are responsible for the following *emotional reactions*:
   • the **trigeminal** (cranial nerve V) and **facial** (cranial nerve VII) nuclei, which control the muscles of facial expression during emotions such as fear;
   • the nuclei of the **periaqueductal grey** (**PAG**) area, which cause four main responses, those of *freeze reaction* (i.e. behavioural arrest), *defensive* and *predatory aggression* and *flight from danger*, depending on which part is stimulated;
   • the **nucleus reticularis pontis caudalis**, which causes a startled response;

- the **dorsal lateral tegmental** nucleus, which activates the higher centres of the cortex onto full alert;
- the **locus ceruleus** nucleus, which increases cortical vigilance through noradrenergic pathways;
- the nuclei of the **ventral tegmental area**, which increases behavioural arousal through dopaminergic pathways and mediates for offensive aggression.

See page 187

See page 114
See page 148

2 Various nuclei of the **hypothalamus**, which are responsible for the following *physical responses*:
- the **periventricular group** of nuclei, which causes increased *sympathetic nervous system* activity;
- various nuclei which together influence the release of stress-related *hormones* into the blood.

See page 18

The neurobiology of emotions is now becoming clearer as research unpicks the delicate nerve networks that link the various components of the brain.

The biology of stress

As a subject, stress is assuming much importance in everyday life, with many articles being published on aspects such as stress in the workplace and **post-traumatic stress disorder**. Stress is both a physical and a mental phenomenon, and an examination of the physiological processes it causes emphasises the harm that excessive or long-term stress can do.

Stressors – adverse environmental factors causing stress – cause undesirable stimuli to enter the thalamus of the brain via the sensory nervous system. Using the emotional pathways shown in Figures 7.2 and 7.3, the stress stimuli pass through the amygdala and on to the hypothalamus. The hypothalamic neuroendocrine response occurs, causing a number of physical changes:

- The autonomic nervous system switches to *sympathetic* activation and this causes the heart rate, blood pressure and blood sugar to rise. The hormone **adrenaline** is secreted into the blood from the **adrenal medulla** by direct stimulation from the sympathetic nervous system. This has the effect of augmenting the sympathetic activity, pushing up the blood pressure and heart rate further. The other hormone released into the blood from the adrenal medulla is **noradrenaline**, which diverts blood away from the skin to supply to the brain and muscles. This may be essential for a quick retreat from the stressor.
- The endocrine component of the hypothalamus releases **corticotropin-releasing factor** or hormone (**CRF** or **CRH**), which causes the release of **adrenocorticotropic hormone** (**ACTH**) from the anterior lobe of the pituitary gland into the general circulation. This in turn causes the release of **cortisol** from the adrenal cortex. The blood level of cortisol then rises, a well-known physical response to stress. In fact, the rise in blood cortisol level is so significant in stress that it has been suggested to measure cortisol levels as a way of measuring stress itself. Cortisol binds

See page 10

to receptors in the cytoplasm of many neurons and causes **gene transcription** (activation of genes) leading to **protein synthesis**. The production of proteins is, in the short term, protective to nerve cells. One effect is to increase the influx of calcium (Ca^{2+}) into the neurons and this improves neuronal function. Cortisol also activates the brain so that it can cope better with new experiences; it causes increased blood glucose levels by mobilising energy stores and these together improve the brain's ability to learn. However, higher levels of cortisol in stressed children can damage their mental ability, causing withdrawn, shy behaviour associated with increased physical ill health, while the child becomes more easily upset.

CRF is itself generating a lot of interest amongst researchers because high CRF levels are now implicated in a number of neuropsychiatric conditions, including anorexia nervosa, anxiety and depression, and more is said about the last in Chapter 9. A low CRF level is also involved in neurodegerative disorders such as Alzheimer's disease. Two CRF receptors have been isolated, CRF1 and CRF2, which bind the hormone in the pituitary gland, in several parts of the brain and, somewhat surprisingly, in the spleen. Stress normally causes a down-regulation of the number of CRF receptors in the anterior pituitary. In chronic stress, this down-regulation may be insufficient or simply fail, and a future generation of drugs designed to block CRF receptors is under development to help relieve the symptoms of chronic stress.

Components of the immune system become involved in the stress response, a process studied under the title **psychoneuroimmunology**. Stress causes changes to the immune system, in particular **immunosuppression**, a reduction in the immune response which increases the risk of infection. **Natural killer** (**NK**) **cells** (those that kill virally infected and malignant cells), **lymphocytes** (the main cells of the immune system) and an antibody called **immunoglobulin A** (**IgA**) are all significantly reduced in stress. These responses suggest that brain neuromodulators released during stress have a wide influence over body functions both inside and outside of the nervous system (Kaye *et al.* 2000).

The symptoms of stress are pallor, raised pulse rate and blood pressure, deeper respiration, sweating, dilated pupils, nausea, frequency of urination and restlessness. Many of these can be recognised at 'side-effects' of the neuroendocrine response; the sweating, for example, is due to sympathetic activity, and the same system combined with adrenaline also drives up the blood pressure and increases the heart rate. This response is a compensatory mechanism brought into play by the body to correct the physiological changes, which would otherwise cause the blood pressure to fall in stress.

In the long term, when stress is persistent for months or years, the result is different. Chronic stress causes many complications, including possible premature ageing of the brain with neuronal losses. The hippocampus is the most likely candidate for cellular losses due to chronic stress. Other long-term effects of chronic cortisol release during stress include **hypertension** (high blood pressure), **peptic ulceration** (ulcers of the stomach and duodenum), depression, substance abuse and anxiety.

Stress and child abuse

Stress occurring during childhood causes 'a cascade of molecular and neuro-biological effects that irreversibly alter neural development' (Teicher 2002). Such stress is the result of child abuse, either active (physical beatings or sexual abuse) or passive (neglect or isolation). In each case the brain is exposed to extensive fear, and permanent damage often results from this type of stress. The damage includes:

- irregularities in the function of the left frontal and temporal lobes of the cerebrum;
- reduced size of the hippocampus and amygdala, again most often seen on the left side of the brain;
- abnormalities within the cerebellar vermis.

The hippocampus continues its development beyond birth, well into childhood, and is one of the few areas of the brain where neurons continue to grow after birth. New neurons form new synaptic connections, and it is these neurons and their connections that are disrupted permanently when subjected to the extreme fear of abuse. In the amygdala, the $GABA_A$ receptor is significantly altered by the severe fear accompanying abuse, causing a loss of its inhibitory function. The result is excessive stimulation of the limbic system (called **limbic irritability**), i.e. abnormal excessive function of the area that governs emotions.

The cerebellar vermis (the central ridge between the cerebellar hemispheres, see Figure 5.10) is another area that continues growing and developing new neurons after birth. The vermis has some control over noradrenaline and dopamine release within the brain stem. Vermis abnormalities (now being linked to several mental disorders including depression, schizophrenia and autism) may push these neurotransmitters into imbalance. Activation and dominance of the dopamine system is linked with increased attention in the *left* hemisphere; activation and dominance of the noradrenaline system is linked with increased attention in the *right* hemisphere. Developmental abnormalities occurring in the vermis after birth as a result if the stress of child abuse may be the cause of the left lateral defects observed in the cerebral and limbic areas. The results of such damage are depression, withdrawal, suicidal tendencies, anxiety, anger, aggression, delinquency, unstable relationships and personality disorders, any of which can occur at any point later in life. Teicher (2002) summarised the studies by saying:

Society reaps what it sows in the way it nurtures its children. Stress sculpts the brain to exhibit various antisocial . . . behaviours. . . . Stress can permanently wire a child's brain to cope with a malevolent world. . . . Our stark conclusion is that we see the need to do much more to ensure that child abuse does not happen in the first place, because once these key brain alterations occur, there may be no going back.

(Teicher 2002)

Post-traumatic stress disorder

Post-traumatic stress disorder (**PTSD**) is a stress condition that occurs in some people exposed to a severe traumatic incident, such as a train crash, either as a survivor or as a rescuer. The environmental incident that triggers the stress clearly has some major effect on brain function, involving changes in the neurochemistry. The pathway that links the hypothalamus to the pituitary, and on to the adrenal gland (the CRF → ACTH → cortisol route) is severely affected, resulting in low cortisol release into the blood (the opposite of acute stress) and therefore a compensatory increase in cortisol receptor sensitivity. In the brain, serotonin and noradrenaline activities are increased, both of which are involved in memory retrieval, and the hippocampus is enlarged. Since the hippocampus is a site of memory function, these changes may account for the number and frequency of **flashbacks** these people suffer, where the original sights, sounds and smells of the incident are relived, often many times, for months or years after the event. This constant re-enactment of the incident is a trauma in itself, seriously disturbing the lifestyle of those who suffer from it. It may require several years of therapy and sensitive understanding on the part of nurses to achieve an outcome that improves the quality of life for those who suffer from this problem (Deahl 1996).

Rosenzweig *et al.* (1999) reported studies done on American Vietnam war veterans with PTSD who suffered from memory changes (e.g. **amnesia** of some traumatic events), flashbacks and problems with short-term memory. They showed an 8% reduction in the size of the hippocampus, but no other structural abnormality. There also appeared to be a genetic susceptibility involved, making some more vulnerable to the effects of trauma than others.

The emotions of life experiences

The neuroanatomy and physiology of the many possible human emotions have fascinated neuroscientists for a long time. Here, we consider some of these emotions and what little we know of their neurological basis:

Religious experiences occur when a subject becomes aware of a sense of an almighty power in their presence, which they usually called God, and may sometimes experience what they call Heaven. In some people this has changed their lives and they have become ministers of various churches and preach or administer healing powers to others. Neuroscientists go to some lengths to point out that while they have no wish to attempt to disprove the existence of God, they have found that specific types of stimulation of the **temporal lobes** of the cerebrum and the limbic system can generate what can be an overwhelming religious feeling. This is usually coupled with a release of endogenous opiates, which intensifies the experience.

See page 56

Love is an experience most people go through at some point in their lives. Scans of the brains of volunteers taken during the intensified mental emotions of love reveal four main areas of increased brain activity: the **anterior cingulate cortex** (see Figures 7.4, 8.1), the **medial insula** (part of the

143

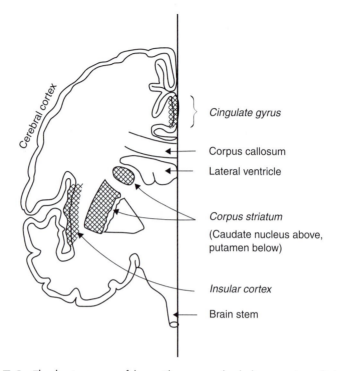

Cingulate gyrus

Corpus callosum

Lateral ventricle

Corpus striatum
(Caudate nucleus above,
putamen below)

Insular cortex

Brain stem

FIGURE 7.4 The brain areas of love. The areas shaded are activated during the emotional feelings of love.

See page 11

cerebral cortex hidden from the surface), and two areas of the **corpus striatum** (part of the basal ganglia) (Figure 7.4) (Phillips 2000a).

Music has attracted much interest from neuroscientists for several reasons. Notably, musical ability is often associated with being a genius and what makes a genius is of great interest to many people. Music has therapeutic properties and for many years has been used as a psychological therapy (*music therapy*). Finally, music generates some of the most intense emotions in some people, anything from excitement to depression, and the question is *why?*

This question remains unanswered, but some interesting concepts point the way. Music has a lot to do with *motion*, and motion has a lot to do with *emotion* (the two words have a common origin, i.e. *motum* = movement). Indeed, the separate sections of a symphony are called movements. Specific emotions, such as love or fear, have definite signs which we can identify in each other and can respond to and take forward. Tonal music also has specific signatures that we can pick out and relate to, like a rhythm or a tune, and music is rarely static, it is constantly driving forward. So music and emotions have very similar components. Just as one angry or laughing person can make others angry or laugh, so music performed by one person can engender emotional moods in an audience. The parts of the brain involved in music appreciation are slowly being revealed. Scans have shown a distinct response from the right temporal lobe of the cerebrum when exposed to tonal music. This is part of the conscious brain and its activation should be no surprise, since the temporal lobe is involved in both hearing and personality. But below this level of the brain, the subconscious areas involved in emotion are also contributing to the response to music. Since sound is one of the earliest experiences we have, even while still in the uterus, the sounds of pitch and rhythm affect our neurological development from the start of life. Neuroscientists believe that the corpus callosum is involved in the mother–child relationship, of which sound is a major part, and the corpus callosum, along with the limbic system, is associated with emotion (Robertson 1996). Another unusual observation is the appearance of bizarre musical hallucinations in patients who have had damage to the dorsal part of the **pons** (part of the brain stem). The music they hear is in keeping with the style of music that is already familiar to them, as though a musical memory is unlocked and floods out into the conscious brain. Perhaps the damage has removed certain inhibitory pathways, allowing the music to be heard.

See page 15

A lot of speculation revolves around whether musical ability is genetic, and therefore runs in families. The composer Mozart was taught by a musical father and other famous composers such as Bach and Johann Strauss also had musical offspring. Now scientists have identified that several genes are involved in the musical ability of both parents and their offspring. Genes are thought to control the function of several sites in the brain that determine **pitch perception**, the ability to recognise different notes. Pitch and rhythm are reported as left hemisphere functions, while the right hemisphere works on melody and timbre (the tone quality of an instrument). Indeed, a part of the temporal lobe called the **planus temporale** (see also Williams syndrome) is normally bigger on the left than the right, but is bigger still on the left in those persons with perfect pitch (Figure 5.12). Children with pitch control genes that are active from an early age can progress quickly with music, while others without these genes may progress more slowly or abandon music in favour of other pursuits.

See page 85

More research needs to be done before we can fully explain why **music therapy** is good for the disturbed mind. Playing Mozart (e.g. Sonata K448) to epileptic patients has reduced the incidence of epileptic fits (Jenkins and Murray 2001), and music played to dementia patients has improved their communication and spatial skills. This phenomenon has been called the **Mozart effect** (Kliewer 1999).

Ghosts, phantoms and doppelgangers may have a neurological basis. The phenomenon of **phantom limb** (i.e. the feeling that an amputated limb is still present) has been a problem for years. Certain cells in the somatic sensory cortex that receive sensations from that limb find they no longer have an input because the limb is gone. They are redundant cells, but they are still alive and may generate their own random impulses which then trick the brain into thinking that the limb is still present. Perhaps the doppelgangers (identical copies of a person, often called 'doubles'), which are seen by that same person, or by someone else, have a similar cause; the phantom limb is elaborated to become the entire body. 'Out of body' experiences and ghosts could also be phantom copies of the body generated by the cerebral cortex, 'seen' by the *mind* rather than the eye and interpreted as an external image (Phillips 2000b). One good example of this is the case of a man driving his van to work who passed *himself* driving exactly the same van in the opposite direction. Both *he* and *himself* stared at each other in amazement as they drove past. For such an event to occur in reality is impossible, and a mental image of himself, generated by his own brain and 'seen' by the mind as an external image, is the best explanation we have at present. The fact that neither 'person' stopped, got out or spoke to the other (i.e. the obvious thing to do) suggests that physical evidence of the other person being real was probably unobtainable, indirectly supporting the brain image theory. Other cases of 'out of body' experiences (called **depersonalisation**), such as the patient who felt as though *he* (his conscious self) was about one meter in front of *himself* (his physical body) all the time, can cause a great deal of distress and may require some form of 'therapy' and very sensitive nursing care.

Anxiety disorders

See page 155

Anxiety is a major psychological problem to which there is no easy solution. Drugs can alleviate the symptoms (see *anxiolytic drugs*) and make life more tolerable for the patient, but they are not a cure. Anxiety appears to involve the amygdala, where cholecystokinin (CCK) receptors are found, and an increase in the level of this hormone in the amygdala will generate a bout of anxiety. The psychological symptoms of anxiety include a sense of fear or apprehension, restlessness and irritability, loss of concentration and disturbed sleep. The physical symptoms include sweating, pallor, palpitations, dry mouth, numbness, dizziness and fainting, frequency of micturition, difficulty in swallowing, shortness of breath and tightness of the chest, perhaps with chest pain. There are four categories of anxiety disorder: **general anxiety disorder** (a category of patients fail to meet the criteria for any of the other three conditions in this group), **panic attacks**, **phobias** and **obsessive-compulsive disorder** (Peveler and Baldwin 1996).

Fear, aggression and phobic states

Fear

Fear is potentially a useful attribute since its presence is a warning that something is hazardous and should be avoided, and this can save lives. But fear is a double-edged sword, a phenomenon that can be either exciting or destructive in people's lives. As an excitement, people seek fear for recreational purposes (roller-coaster rides or horror movies); but as a destructive mechanism, fear keeps people at home and prevents them from getting on with their lives. Neuroscientists are keen to understand the anatomy and physiology of fear so as to be able to unlock the prison in which so many frightened people spend their lives.

Three brain components appear to be communicating during periods of fear brought about by a potentially threatening environmental stimulus:

- The prefrontal cortex of the cerebrum, which, along with the tip of the temporal lobe, assesses the stimulus for the potential as a threat to life. These two areas are often collectively called the **neocortex**.
- The amygdala, which adds the emotional dimension to the experience of fear.
- The hypothalamus, which sets in motion the **hypathalamo–pituitary–adrenal axis** (i.e. the CRF → ACTH → cortisol route).

See page 66

The importance of the temporal lobe and amygdala in the creation of fear is illustrated in the **Kluver–Bucy syndrome**. This condition is caused by a lesion of the temporal lobes, apparently extending into the amygdala below. Such a lesion may be the result of a stroke or a head injury or may be associated with epilepsy or dementia, and brings about a general blunting of emotions coupled with a profound loss of fear. Five distinct behavioural symptoms are characteristic of the disorder:

- **Psychic blindness**, an inability to recognise common objects and what they represent, despite normal vision.
- Oral tendencies, where all such objects are 'tested' by being put in the mouth. This leads to the concept that these patients eat everything, but more probably they are using the mouth as a mechanism of sensory input to aid recognition.
- **Hypermetamorphosis**, an overwhelming compulsion to explore everything in the immediate environment.
- Increased sexual tendencies, including making inappropriate sexual advances to others, even inanimate objects.
- Emotional blunting (known as **flattening of affect**), with a profound loss of all sense of fear.

The hormones released during fear are basically **adrenaline** (released into the blood and circulated to all parts of the body) and **endorphins** (released into the central nervous system). These help the brain to cope with the stress that accompanies the fear; adrenaline promotes the sympathetic response and endorphins help to protect the brain from excessive stress stimuli. After the experience of fear is over, the hormone **dopamine** is released into the brain, giving the mind a sense of joy, well-being and the satisfaction of achievement (similar to the feelings achieved by increased dopamine as a consequence of drug abuse; see Chapter 4). The *feel-good factor* created by dopamine is probably the reason why some people seek out excitement. The dopamine receptor known as D_4 appears to be involved, and this receptor is coded for by a gene on chromosome 11 (the **D4DR** gene). However, there appear to be two forms of this gene: *long* and *short*. Those who have inherited the slightly longer form of the gene are more resistant to dopamine, and therefore need additional dopamine to have the feel-good effect that they call a *buzz*. These people have to take extra risks to obtain more dopamine, and therefore they seek out adventurous and risky activities. For those with the shorter version of the gene such risks are unnecessary and appear foolhardy.

See page 56

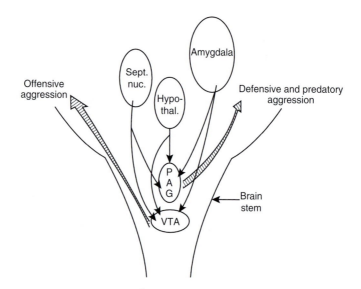

FIGURE 7.5 Aggression. Inputs from the septal nucleus (Sept. nuc.) and amygdala to the periaquaductal grey (PAG) cause defensive and predatory aggression; inputs to the ventral tegmental area (VTA) cause offensive aggression.

Aggression

Aggression (Figure 7.5) takes three main forms: *offensive* (against another person), *defensive* (protecting against attack) and *predatory* (seeking satisfaction from others for a need such as food). The neurochemistry of this phenomenon is strongly linked to the levels of serotonin in the brain. All the evidence indicates that serotonin has a calming effect on an individual, calming impulsive behaviour in particular, and therefore aggression is linked to low levels of serotonin. Reduced levels of serotonin correlate particularly *See page 183* well with aggression to oneself (i.e. suicide) and with impulsive aggression towards others (Coccaro 1995). Corresponding changes in serotonin receptors, consistent with serotonin receptor structural abnormalities, have been found in the frontal lobes of those committing violent suicide. The poor function of the serotonin system may be due to an error in the gene that codes for *See page 47* **tryptophan hydroxylase**, a key enzyme in the synthesis of serotonin.

The areas of the brain involved are also becoming apparent. Offensive aggression appears to be mediated through the **ventral tegmental area** *See page 114* (**VTA**) in the brain stem, while different parts of the **periaquaductal grey** *See page 139* (**PAG**) are associated with defensive and predatory aggression. These areas are themselves moderated by inputs from the hypothalamus, the septum and the amygdala (Figure 7.5). Examples of this are defensive and predatory aggression. Defensive aggression can be activated by stimulation of the medial hypothalamus, while predatory aggression can be activated by stimulation of the lateral hypothalamus.

Other hormones are involved in mediating aggression, notably the **androgens**, especially **testosterone**. Exposure of the fetus to testosterone *See page 71* causes masculinisation of the brain (**prenatal androgenisation**), and at puberty further exposure causes males to increase their aggressive tendencies. The effect of androgens on aggression between males appears to be mediated through another part of the hypothalamus called the **pre-optic area**. While testosterone is significantly lower in females, some women receive exposure to higher levels than others, and the women thus exposed, either as a fetus or later in life, show increased aggressive tendencies towards others. Pregnant women with higher testosterone levels than average are more likely to have daughters described as *tomboys*, i.e. interested in male-, rather than female-orientated toys and games. The opposite also appears to be true, with higher-estrogen mothers having daughters with very feminine ways. Estradiol, the main female estrogen, causes a reduction in aggression and a general calming effect on the brain. It is possible that hormonal shifts which result in a lowering of estradiol just prior to menstruation may have some bearing on the **premenstrual syndrome**, a state of irritability and increased aggression that occurs a few days before a menstrual period.

Murder, especially *serial murder*, is a form of offensive aggression that has also sparked a great deal of interest. Neuroscientists want to be able to answer the question: *What goes on inside a serial killer's mind?* Now some answers are coming to light. Murderers appear to lack the level of **prefrontal lobe** activity seen in law-abiding subjects. In the absence of prefrontal lobe activity, the emotions are unmodified in any way by conscious reasoning. Some work carried out on male murderers has shown an actual loss of prefrontal neurons, particularly those neurons responsible for learned remorse, conscience and social sensitivity. These men have been categorised as suffering from **aggressive impulse personality disorder**, or **antisocial personality disorder** (**APD**) (Carlson 2001). Flood (1999) gives an account of the nature and management of personality disorders. APD is characterised by deceitfulness, lack of emotion, life-long antisocial behaviour and irresponsibility. The kind of neuronal loss seen in APD and the characteristics it causes raise issues such as: *Can murderers be held responsible for their crimes if they are missing cells from their brain?* or, *If there is no cure from their brain disorder, should murderers ever be released from custody?* (Ahuja 2002). Murderers also show altered levels of chemicals in the brain. Testosterone appears to be the fuel that drives predetermined behaviour in men. That predetermined behaviour pattern is probably controlled by other factors such as genetics. If the behaviour pattern involves aggression, high levels of testosterone can drive the aggression to the point of murder. Alarmingly high levels of testosterone in some men have been associated with violence involving the rape and murder of women, sometimes multiple women, a problem called **sexual sadism**. The neurotransmitter serotonin normally has an inhibitory effect on such violent behaviour. Killers often have low levels of serotonin, and the combination of high testosterone with low serotonin becomes an explosive mixture that can result in particularly nasty impulsive violent murders that may be repeated several times. Low serotonin in an adult appears to be associated with disruption of the family during that person's childhood. Separation of the child from the mother is the key disrupting factor. Bonding of the child with its mother appears to *mould the mind*, providing stimulus for synaptic connections within the serotonergic pathways of the brain.

Without this maternal love and support, the brain becomes devoid of vital serotonergic pathways and the effects of serotonin remain low.

Some murderers also have high levels of a substance called **cryptopyrol**, a chemical normally found in the liver and obtained from the breakdown of **erythrocytes** (red blood cells). Increased levels of cryptopyrol have a similar activity in the brain to that seen in use of the drug LSD. LSD has the effect of a hallucinogen, i.e. distorting the sensory systems, causing the subject to see the world as a jumble of sensory inputs. *Cannibalistic* behaviour, which is rare, may be simply a response to the need for food in a situation where there is a risk of starvation. Cannibalistic tendencies have been associated with some modern murders and evidence of cannibalistic practices has recently been found in some ancient archaeological sites (McKie 1998). Cannibalism may be caused by physical damage to the frontal lobes, possible from a head injury. It does not seem likely at present that any of this neuroscientific 'evidence' creates the grounds for excusing the perpetrators of their crime by claiming they are 'sick' (Ahuja 2002).

See page 130

Nurses need to be able to manage aggression effectively for their own safety and the safety of others, particularly children, who are unable to protect themselves. Aggression in the public arena and in the workplace is now an escalating problem, and nurses are in the front line for physical and verbal abuse. Sheffield University's **CASE de-escalation model** for coping with a potentially violent situation is an interactive CD-ROM programme for the education of health-care workers. Walker *et al.* (2002) describes the CASE (Calming, Assessing, Self, Enabling) de-escalation model and gives instructions on the prevention and safe management of aggressive situations. Much aggression and violence is associated with excessive consumption of alcohol and drugs, and this complicates the situation. The emphasis must be placed on personal safety and getting help at the earliest opportunity.

Phobias and obsessions

A **phobia** is an irrational fear centred on a specific situation or object, which dominates the lifestyle of the sufferer. We all fear something, but when that fear severely disturbs our waking hours to the point of distorting our life-style it becomes pathological. There are many common phobias, e.g. fear of an *object* such as a spider (**arachnophobia**) or a *situation* such as an enclosed space (**claustrophobia**), but if the person concerned avoids the cause of the phobia as much as possible, they can continue a normal life. Pathological phobic states, however, incapacitate the patient and require medical inter-vention to re-establish a reasonable quality of life.

Obsessions are repeated thoughts, ideas or phrases, and **compulsions** are irresistible repetitive activities, such as repeated hand-washing, which the patient must go through in order to prevent some degree of anxiety. Both of these together in the same patient make up **obsessive-compulsive disorder** (**OCD**). If these activities are stopped or prevented in some way, the person concerned may quickly go into a **panic attack**.

There is some evidence to suggest that both *panic attacks* and *obsessive-compulsive disorder* carry a genetic susceptibility, as a higher than average incidence of such attacks can be demonstrated in some families. It has also been found that an injection of **lactic acid** will cause some individuals to have a panic attack whereas the same injection has no such effect on others, and this suggests that some individuals are genetically more susceptible to panic attacks than others (Maier 1999). Temporal lobe abnormalities have been found in association with anxiety states and panic attacks. It seems that the greater the abnormality, the younger the age of onset of the anxiety (Rosenzweig *et al*. 1999). Reduced frontal lobe activity is also implicated in panic attacks. In the case of both frontal and temporal lobes, a diminished level of activity causes the attack, suggesting that the role of these lobes in understanding and rationalising sensory stimuli is reduced, leaving the limbic system to respond independently. There may be an abnormally raised level of serotonin (5-HT) and abnormal levels of cholecystokinin (CCK) in this disorder, although exactly how they influence the condition is not fully known.

See page 53

Obsessive-compulsive disorder is associated with increased activity of several brain areas, notably the orbitofrontal cortex, the cingulate cortex and the caudate nucleus. Neurosurgery has been used successfully to reduce the symptoms of OCD by cutting through some of the pathways that pass from the frontal lobe to the limbic parts of the brain (Ron 1999). With regard to the caudate nucleus, this part of the basal ganglia receives input from the cerebral cortex and feeds back to the cortex via the thalamus. Two pathways connect it with the thalamus, an excitatory pathway and an inhibitory pathway (Figure 7.6). The former is said to facilitate previously learned and automatic behaviour, while the latter reduces it, thereby allowing the individual to move on to new behaviours. It is suggested that in OCD the excitatory pathway may be overactive, an imbalance that keeps the patient locked in a cycle of repetitive behaviour (Carlson 2001).

An alternative view is that the link between the thalamus and the cortex, including the reciprocal feedback loop from the cortex to the thalamus, has become inhibited, i.e. have become deactivated, for some unknown reason (Clayton 2000). This problem may also be implicated in the cause of depression and the hallucinations suffered in schizophrenia. Artificially stimulating the thalamic-cortical loop with an implanted device may improve the symptoms of OCD.

Eating disorders

Several disorders which result in disturbance of normal eating patterns sometimes need psychological support and therapy. The most important of these are **obesity** (excess weight), **anorexia nervosa** (inadequate eating) and **bulimia nervosa** (loss of control of food intake). The sufferer of anorexia nervosa will eat very little, leading to severe weight loss and starvation to the point of death. In contrast, the patient with bulimia nervosa will periodically go on an eating 'binge'. They will eat lots of high-calorie food and then, feeling guilty, cause vomiting and use laxatives to get rid of it. The biological mechanism of normal food control is very complex and as yet not fully understood. Not until recently has there been any clear idea of what is going wrong in anorexia nervosa.

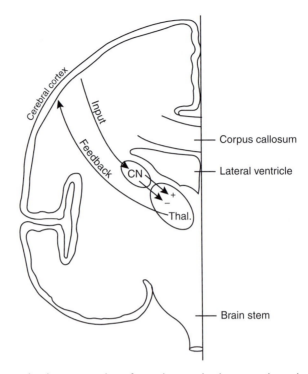

FIGURE 7.6 The loop extending from the cerebral cortex through the caudate nucleus (CN) to the thalamus (Thal.), either excitatory or inhibitory, and back to the cortex, influences learning and automatic behaviour.

Adipose tissue (stored fat under the skin and around internal organs) releases a hormone called **leptin** into the blood (Figure 7.7). This hormone binds to **leptin receptors** in the **arcuate nucleus**, one of the nuclei of the hypothalamus. The binding of leptin to its receptor causes a shut-down of neurons which normally secrete a combination of two proteins, **neuro-peptide Y** (**NPY**) and **agouti-related protein** (**ARP**). Together, these normally act by binding and inhibiting another receptor, the **melanocortin-4 receptor** (**MC-4**). Inhibition of the MC-4 by NYP and ARP in the hypothalamus causes feeding activity, so the blocking of NYP + ARP by leptin stops the individual from feeding. This makes sense when you consider that the greater the mass of adipose tissue the larger the release of leptin; and in circumstances of large adipose mass the need for food should be less. To reinforce this effect, leptin receptors activated by the binding of leptin also stimulate other arcuate neurons, which then release two other proteins called **cocaine and amphetamine regulated transcript** (**CART**) and **α-MSH** (**alpha-melanocyte stimulating hormone**). Together these neuromodulators act on MC-4 receptors to inhibit feeding. So leptin causes *inhibition* of feeding behaviour by *increasing* CART+α-MSH and *decreasing* NYP + ARP (Figure 7.7). What may be happening in anorexia nervosa is that some form of acute stress causes the normal neuroendocrine response, raising blood adrenaline and cortisol levels. This appears

See page 55

See page 65

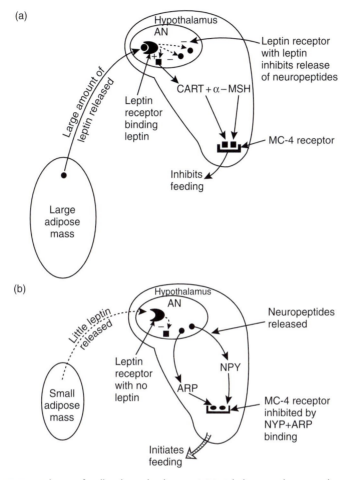

FIGURE 7.7 Adipose feedback to the brain. (a) With large adipose volume, more leptin is released, which binds to leptin receptors in the arcuate nucleus (AN) of the hypothalamus. This causes inhibition of neuropeptide release, but promotes the release of the cocaine and amphetamine regulated transcript (CART) and the alpha-melanocyte stimulating hormone (α-MSH). These bind to MC-4 receptors and inhibit feeding. (b) Little adipose volume releases low levels of leptin; the empty leptin receptor then inhibits the CART/α-MSH release but causes release of neuropeptides. When these bind to MC-4 receptors, feeding is initiated. NPY = neuropeptide Y; ARP = agouti-related protein.

to switch off ARP, just as leptin does, and therefore inhibits feeding. However, once the acute stress is over, the cortisol and adrenaline levels fall to normal, ARP is activated again and feeding behaviour is restored. In anorexia nervosa, the stress is retained in a chronic form (although it may not be recognised as such by the patient or their family), so that high levels of adrenaline and cortisol are retained in the blood. In this way, ARP is continually inhibited, feeding behaviour may be chronically suppressed and the individual will starve. One of the long-term effects of persistent starvation is that the hippocampus shrinks, causing a permanent reduction in the hippocampal role in regulating appetite. Long-term anorexia may cause the type of brain damage that is both irreparable and perpetuates the problem.

Obesity may be due to a reduction in the brain's *sensitivity* to leptin, rather than a reduction in the amount of leptin production. This is possible through several mechanisms:

- The gene for leptin mutates, the changed gene coding for a form of leptin that does not bind to its receptor.
- The gene for the receptor mutates, the changed gene coding for a form of receptor that cannot accept leptin.
- The transporter system that is essential for leptin to cross the blood–brain barrier becomes faulty and less leptin reaches the brain.

Some of these mechanisms have been found in humans, often occurring in families as an inherited trait.

The neurophysiology of eating is further complicated by other control mechanisms. For example, the liver detects levels of blood glucose and fatty acids and signals the brain about these via the vagus nerve (cranial nerve X) (Figure 7.8). The brain area that receives these signals is the **nucleus of the solitary tract** (**NST**) in the brain stem. This nucleus, in turn, relays the information to the lateral hypothalamus. In this way the liver keeps the hypothalamus informed of nutrient levels in circulation. The **lateral hypothalamus** is a major player in the generation of hunger, the **ventromedial**

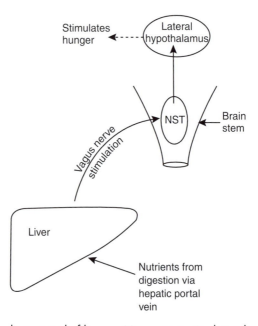

FIGURE 7.8 The liver control of hunger. Vagus nerve stimulation by the liver informs the hypothalamus, via the nucleus of the solitary tract (NST) in the brain stem, about the condition of nutrients in storage. Low nutrient levels may stimulate hunger.

hypothalamus initiating the sensation of **satiety**, i.e. the feeling of fullness. However, most researchers in this subject acknowledge the important regulatory role played by other brain areas, notably the amygdala, the frontal cortex, the substantia nigra and the hippocampus. Some chemicals called **orexins** have been discovered recently, one of which, **orexin A**, is active in the lateral hypothalamus where it promotes an increase in appetite (Carlson 2001). **Orexin B** is active in the sleep–wake cycle. The genetics of obesity may involve the leptin gene mutations mentioned above and the gene for the MC-4 receptor.

To complicate the issue, anorexia nervosa has been associated with abnormally low levels of immune chemicals called **interleukins** (**IL**), notably **IL-2** and **IL-3**, normally produced and released by peripheral white blood cells. The significance of this, including any subsequent effect on the brain, has not yet been fully explored.

If anorexia nervosa really is a *fat phobia*, and *compulsive eating* is a major cause of obesity as has been suggested by some workers in this area, then disorders of this kind may be a distinct subset of anxiety-related disorders. Clearly, much more research is necessary before an effective treatment becomes available.

The anxiolytic drugs

The **benzodiazepines** are a major group of anxiolytic drugs (anxio = anxiety, lytic = dissolving), typified by **diazepam**, and are used widely to reduce levels of anxiety. These drugs bind to the **GABA$_A$** receptor (Figure 3.13) *See page 52* and promote the function of GABA to open the chloride channel that runs through the receptor. In this respect they have a similar action to that of barbiturates and alcohol. The subsequent increase in the influx of chloride into the neuronal postsynaptic membrane causes a greater degree of *resting potential* and blocks any chance of an action potential in that cell. On a widely distributed basis throughout the brain, this drug group has a sedatory effect, i.e. it calms the brain but without inducing sleep (except in high dosage).

Key points

The limbic system

- The limbic system is a series of centres involved in self-preservation and preservation of the species.
- The major components of the limbic system are the amygdala, the mammillary bodies of the hypothalamus, the anterior and dorsal nuclei of the thalamus, several deep nuclei, the septal area, the orbitofrontal cortex of the cerebrum, the hippocampus and parahippocampal gyrus and parts of the temporal lobe.
- The amygdala is the main site for emotions, although emotional states are moderated through several other brain areas as well, notably the frontal and temporal cortex, the hypothalamus and the hippocampus.

- The neuroendocrine response is a normal mechanism adopted by the hypothalamus to combat the effects of stress. It consists of a neurological response via the sympathetic nervous system, and an endocrine response via certain pituitary hormones.

Stress

- Post-traumatic stress disorder (PTSD) is a stress condition that occurs in some people exposed to a severe traumatic incident, such as a train crash. It causes flashbacks, which may be due to the affected CRF → ACTH → cortisol pathway, with low cortisol release into the blood, and an enlarged hippocampus.

Anxiety disorders

- Anxiety appears to involve the amygdala, where increased cholecystokinin (CCK) can cause anxiety.
- There are four categories of anxiety disorder: general anxiety disorder, panic attacks, phobias and obsessive-compulsive disorder.

Fear

- Three brain components appear to be communicating during periods of fear, the prefrontal and temporal cortex, the amygdala and the hypothalamus, involving the hypathalamo–pituitary–adrenal axis, i.e. the CRF → ACTH → cortisol route.
- A lesion of the temporal lobes and the amygdala causes Kluver–Bucy syndrome. It causes psychic blindness, oral tendencies, hypermetamorphosis, increased sexual tendencies and emotional blunting.
- The hormones released during fear are adrenaline and endorphins and, after the experience of fear, dopamine is released.

Aggression

- Aggression takes three main forms: offensive, defensive and predatory.
- Aggression is linked to serotonin levels in the brain, i.e. serotonin has a calming effect.
- Testosterone increases aggression whereas estrogen calms the brain.
- Offensive aggression involves the ventral tegmental area (VTA) in the brain stem, whereas the periaquaductal grey (PAG) is associated with defensive and predatory aggression.

Phobias and obsessive-compulsive disorder

- A phobia is an irrational fear centred on a specific situation or object.
- Obsessions are repeated thoughts, ideas or phrases; compulsions are irresistible repetitive activities.
- Reduced frontal lobe activity is implicated in panic attacks.

- Obsessive-compulsive disorder is associated with increased activity of the orbitofrontal cortex, the cingulate cortex and the caudate nucleus.
- Possibly, the excitatory pathway that connects the caudate nucleus with the thalamus is overactive in OCD, causing an imbalance where excitation exceeds inhibition.

Eating disorders

- The lateral hypothalamus is the main component that causes hunger, the ventromedial hypothalamus initiating the sensation of satiety.
- The most important of the eating disorders are obesity, anorexia nervosa and bulimia nervosa.
- In anorexia nervosa, chronic stress may cause high adrenaline and cortisol to remain in the blood, inhibiting ARP and feeding, leading to starvation.
- Obesity may be due to a reduction in the brain's sensitivity to leptin.
- The anxiolytics bind to the $GABA_A$ receptor and promote GABA to open the chloride channel, causing inhibition of action potentials and calming of the brain.

References

Ahuja A. (2002) Bad brain or bad person? *The Times* (T2 Science) 22 April: 10.

Carlson N. R. (2001) *Physiology of Behavior*. Allyn and Bacon, Boston.

Clayton J. (2000) Caught napping. *New Scientist*, **165** (2227): 42–45.

Coccaro E. F. (1995) The biology of aggression. *Scientific American: Science and Medicine*, Jan/Feb 1995: 38–47.

Deahl M. P. (1996) Post-traumatic stress syndrome. *Medicine*, **24** (2): 15–16.

Flood G. (1999) What are personality disorders and are they treatable? *British Journal of Nursing*, **8** (4): 231–234.

Jenkins J. and Murray C. S. (2001) Mozart 'can cut epilepsy'. http://news.bbc.co.uk/hi/english/health/newsid_1251000/1251839.stm

Kaye J., Morton J., Bowcutt M. and Maupin D. (2000) Stress, depression and psychneuroimmunology. *Journal of Neuroscience Nursing*, **32** (2): 93–100.

Kliewer G. (1999) The Mozart effect. *New Scientist*, **164** (2211; 6 Nov): 34–37.

McKie R. (1998) The people eaters. *New Scientist*, **157** (2125): 43–46.

Maier M. (1999) Magnetic resonance spectroscopy in neuropsychiatry, *in* Ron M. A. and David A. S. (eds), *Disorders of Brain and Mind*. Cambridge University Press, Cambridge.

Peveler R. and Baldwin D. (1996) Anxiety disorders. *Medicine*, **24** (2): 11–14.

Phillips H. (2000a) So you think your're in love? *New Scientist*, 8 July: 11.

Phillips H. (2000b) Mind phantoms. *New Scientist*, 8 July: 11.

Robertson P. (1996) *Music and the Mind*. Channel 4 Television publication.

Ron M. A. (1999) Psychiatric manifestations of demonstrable brain disease, *in* Ron M. A. and David A. S. (eds), *Disorders of Brain and Mind*. Cambridge University Press, Cambridge.

Rosenzweig M. R., Leiman A. L. and Breedlove S. M. (1999) *Biological Psychology: An Introduction to Behavioral, Cognitive, and Clinical Neuroscience*. Sinauer Associates, Sunderland, MA.

Teicher M. H. (2002) The neurobiology of child abuse. *Scientific American*, **286** (3; March): 54–61.

Walker J., Wren J. and Skalycz A. (2002) Safety first. *Nursing Times*, **98** (9; 28 Feb): 20–21.

Chapter 8

Schizophrenia

- Introduction
- The genetic influence in schizophrenia
- Brain pathology
- Neurodevelopment as a factor
- The biochemical changes in schizophrenia
- The possible role of environmental factors
- The antipsychotic drugs
- Key points

Introduction

A student of psychiatric nursing in the 1960s would have had a classroom session on schizophrenia possibly consisting of a description of the symptoms and types of the disease, with mention of the drugs used at the time to treat the condition. Hardly anything would have been said about what was happening in the brain, simply because very little was known then about the biology of the disease. Much progress had been made by the 1960s, of course, to dispel the pre-Victorian notion that this disorder was due to devils in the brain, but the emphasis was placed on the psychology of the condition rather than any physical disorder. Now, however, the evidence is mounting that there is an organic cause to schizophrenia, and much intense research is now being conducted in a major effort to solve this mind-destroying problem.

Schizophrenia is a major psychotic illness causing a series of symptoms that rob the patient of their cognitive thought, their socialisation skills and ultimately their personality. These symptoms fall into two categories, positive and negative (Table 8.1). These two groups of symptoms may indicate that the term 'schizophrenia' is being used to describe an amalgamation of two distinct syndromes, one demonstrating a predominance of positive symptoms (type I), the other a predominance of negative symptoms (type II) (Yakeley and Murray 1996). The relationship between the two syndromes is interesting: delays in the early neurodevelopment of an individual have been correlated with negative symptoms, disturbance of language and attention, and poor social adjustment later in life. The negative symptoms are usually resistant to all attempts to prevent them as they may be the consequence of irreversible brain damage (see brain cell losses) (Carlson 2001) and, in young people, this indicates a poor outcome. Positive symptoms such as hallucinations and delusions, on the other hand, tend to occur a little later in life, as the disorder becomes more advanced. They are probably due to increased activity in the dopamine and possibly the noradrenaline brain circuits (Carlson 2001). It seems that negative symptoms, language plus attention problems and social maladjustment are also symptoms of affective disorder (see Chapter 9), but if you add positive symptoms to this scenario it becomes schizophrenia. If this *two-syndrome hypothesis* turns out to be correct, it will have implications for the treatment and management of schizophrenia. The management of schizophrenic symptoms provides a major challenge for nurses caring for these clients. Symptoms such as hallucinations and delusions are hard to comprehend and manage successfully (Holland *et al.* 1999).

Although at the moment the cause of schizophrenia is still unknown, there is a huge and growing volume of biological data concerning the disease, much of which still needs to be fitted together, to explain the symptoms. It does now appear, however, that a number of factors act together to influence the onset of schizophrenia. This chapter provides an account of the known biological aspects of the disease and how they may be affecting brain function.

The risk of developing schizophrenia is about 1% for the population of the world as a whole; that is, 1 in 100 persons will develop the disease on average. The age of onset of symptoms is mostly later in women than in men; males usually begin showing evidence of the disease in their teens or early twenties (around 15–25 years).

The genetic influence in schizophrenia

The evidence strongly implicates a genetic component in the cause of schizophrenia (Taylor 1999), and some specific genes have been found that may play a part in the cause. The disease is probably **polygenic** (several genes involved interacting with environmental factors). The suggestion of gene involvement is based on studies of monozygotic (identical) twins, who have close to 100% of their genes in common between them, and other family groups involved in schizophrenia. Table 8.2 shows the concordance rate, i.e. the percentage chance of related members of the family developing the disease.

If one of a set of monozygotic twins develops schizophrenia, the other twin has a 40–50% chance of having the disease, which is clearly much

TABLE 8.1 The symptoms of schizophrenia

Symptom	Types	Explanation, examples
Positive symptoms Those unwanted aspects that the patient would prefer to do without;? caused by increased dopamine activity. Usually associated with abrupt onset of the disease.		
Thought disorder *includes* **Delusions** (disorder of thought content) (Holland *et al.* 1999)	Ideas of reference	Ordinary items have special meaning for the patient, e.g. 'Three milk bottles delivered today means I have three days to live'
	Concrete thinking	Everything is literal, no abstract thinking, e.g. 'I must fly' means to the patient you will grow wings and take to the air
	Flights of ideas	Rapid, uncontrolled thoughts passing quickly from one to another
	Grandeur	False belief of great status or importance, e.g. 'I own the hospital'
	Paranoia	False belief that harm is directed to the patient, e.g. 'Next door's TV is beaming death rays at me'
	Persecution	False belief that people are against the patient, e.g. 'The doctor is killing me with drugs'
	Body	False belief that the body is changed in some way, e.g. 'My head is made of plastic'
Hallucinations (Holland *et al.* 1999)	Tactile	Feeling things that are not there
	Aural	Hearing things that are not there, notable voices talking to them
	Visual	Seeing things that are not there, notably little people
Bizarre behaviour	e.g. catatonia or inappropriate aggression	Long periods of no visible movement. Violent outbursts
Negative symptoms Those attributes taken away from the patient that they would prefer to keep;? caused by neuron losses. Usually associated with gradual onset of the disease.		
Withdrawal from reality	Isolation from the real world into an inner world of the mind	Profound loss of self-care
Loss of volition (or motivation)	The willingness to do things is lost	Remains seated all day if not motivated
Loss (or blunting) of affect	Mood and emotions are lost or inappropriate	Remains emotionless or cries (or laughs) without reason
Loss of speech (or speech content)	Speaks very little	Remains quiet all day

TABLE 8.2 Risk of developing schizophrenia

Family relationship	Genetic risk concordance rate
Monozygotic twins	40–50%
Dizygotic twins	15–17%
A sibling affected	10%
One parent affected	15%
Both parents affected	35%
One parent and one sibling affected	17%

higher than the 1% general population rate. However, given that nearly all their genes are the same, it might be expected that the concordance rate would be close to 100%, such that if one twin acquired the disease the other definitely would. But this difference is the result of environmental factors influencing the course of events, the environment being an important part of all polygenic disorders. Table 8.3 identifies the most important genes thought to influence schizophrenia and what we understand of their function. This list is not exhaustive; other genes appear in the literature from time to time, and no doubt will continue to do so.

The type of **gene error** could be a **fragile site**, a point where the DNA is particularly prone to breakage (fragile sites are especially involved in several mental health disorders, see **fragile X syndrome**). **CAG** or **CGG** repeats are abnormal multiple copies of three nucleotide bases along the DNA, in this case **cytosine–adenine–guanine** and **cytosine–guanine–guanine**, respectively. Repeat sequences are sometimes the cause of disorders of the brain (see Huntington disease). **Polymorphism** is the existence of two or more variants of the gene. *See page 80* *See page 231*

Brain pathology

The pathological changes seen in the schizophrenic patient's brain when compared to normal brains at post mortem are not gross, but some distinct abnormalities have been consistently reported. These include mostly enlarged ventricles, a reduction in brain weight of about 5% and a shortening of the length of the brain. On close study, it can be seen that there are some reductions in the volume (i.e. neuronal losses) within the prefrontal cortex, the insula cortex (part of the cerebrum hidden from view deep at the bottom of the lateral fissure), the entorhinal cortex, the hippocampus and the temporal lobe grey matter. The entorhinal cortex and the anterior hippocampus both suffer losses of about 20% of their neurons. These areas of the brain also apparently show a change in the **cytoarchitecture**, i.e. alterations in the cellular *structure*, not just numbers of cells lost. *See page 164*

Two large areas of the frontal cortex are Brodmann 10 and Brodmann 4 (the primary motor cortex). Brodmann 10 shows significant losses of neurons in cell layer vi, and lower than normal density of the interneurons in

TABLE 8.3 The major genes examined in schizophrenia research. See text for explanations of terms

Gene	Gene locus	Function (if known)	Gene error (if known)	Possible role in schizophrenia
KCNN3 (SK3)	1q21–q22	Calcium-activated potassium channel	CAG repeats	The longer gene may code for a potassium channel with subtle abnormal changes in function, altering neuron activity
DRD3	3q13.3	Codes for dopamine receptor D_3	Polymorphism	Dopamine receptors implicated in the biochemical cause of psychosis
NOTCH4	6p21.3			Highly associated with schizophrenia
ATX1 (ATX = ataxin)	6p23	Codes for the protein ataxin 1		Possibly associated with severity of symptoms
DRD4	11p15.5	Codes for dopamine receptor D_4		Dopamine receptors implicated in the biochemical cause of psychosis
DRD2	11q23	Codes for dopamine receptor D_2	Polymorphism	Dopamine receptors implicated in the biochemical cause of psychosis
5-HT 2A receptor	13q14–q21	Codes for serotonin receptor 2A	Polymorphism	Receptor variation may disturb serotonin pathways from the raphe nucleus

Gene	Location	Function	Variation	Significance
CHRNA7	15q14	Codes for the alpha-7 subunit of the nicotinic acetylcholine receptor	Polymorphism	Nicotinic receptors are involved in the inhibition of sensory stimuli that may be reduced in schizophrenia leading to hallucinations
GNAL	18p	Codes for the G-protein alpha subunit coupled to the D_1 dopamine receptor	Nucleotide repeat sequence	Dopamine receptors implicated in the biochemical cause of psychosis
SCZD4 (SCZ = schizophrenia)	22q11–q13		Deletions within 22q11	Increases susceptibility to schizophrenia
DXYS14	X telomere		Shared alleles in affected siblings	Schizophrenic patients often have excess X chromosomes
5-HT 1A receptor gene	5q11.2–q13	Codes for serotonin receptor		Receptor variation may disturb serotonin pathways from the raphe nucleus
cPLA2 (phospholipase gene)	Chromosome 19	Controls the production of the enzyme cytosolic phospholipase	Diamorphic site	Excess enzyme may cause neuronal phospholipid breakdown in schizophrenia
Type 1 sigma receptor gene	19p13.3	Codes for sigma receptor	Polymorphism	The drug haloperidol binds to sigma receptors

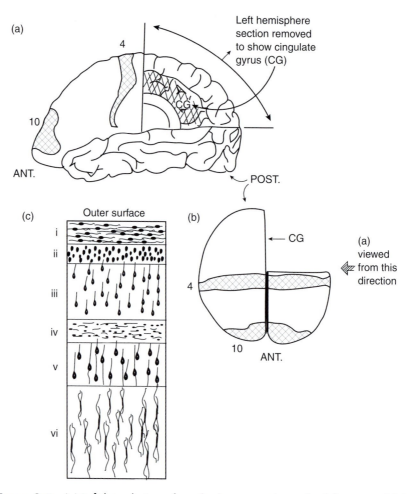

FIGURE 8.1 (a) Left lateral view of cerebral cortex with much of the parietal lobe removed back to the midline to show the cingulate gyrus (CG), and also shows Brodmann areas 4 and 10. (b) Superior view of the same as (a). (c) Section through the cerebral cortex to show the cell layers. The areas identified in (a) and (b) all suffer a loss of cells in schizophrenia. Brodmann 4 and 10 both show cell losses in layer vi, with Brodmann 10 also showing reduced cell density in layer ii. The cingulate gyrus shows cell losses in layer v. ANT. = anterior, POST. = posterior.

layer ii. Brodmann 4 shows significant losses in layer vi. In addition, the cingulate gyrus (Brodmann 24) shows notable numbers of neuronal losses in cell layer v (Figure 8.1).

Cell losses in early-onset schizophrenia have recently been seen on brain scans for the first time (Thompson *et al.* 2001). Over the five-year period from 13 to 18 years of age, 12 schizophrenic patients who were scanned showed brain cell losses progressing from the parietal lobes to many other parts of the brain. This event occurring in the teens would account for the onset of symptoms at that time, probably triggered by an environmental agent. Those with the greatest losses of cells suffered the worst symptoms.

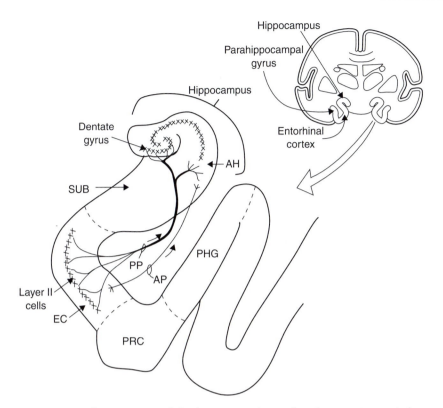

Figure 8.2 Schematic view of the hippocampal complex showing Ammon's horn (AH), subiculum (SUB), entorhinal cortex (EC), perirhinal cortex (PRC) and the parahippocampal gyrus (PHG). PP is the perforant pathway running from layer ii cells of the EC to the AH and dentate gyrus. AP is the alvear pathway running from the EC to the AH. The inset shows a section through the brain with the area involved labelled.

The **entorhinal cortex** (Brodmann area 28) is next to the **parahippocampal gyrus**, which in turn is part of the temporal lobe cortex close to the hippocampus (Figure 8.2). The **subiculum**, which blends directly into **Ammon's horn** of the hippocampus, is sometimes included as part of the hippocampus. The entorhinal cortex is the origin of two main pathways: the **alvear** pathway which goes to Ammon's horn, and the **perforant** pathway which also terminates in Ammon's horn and the **dentate gyrus** (also part of the hippocampal complex). These two pathways form direct communication with the hippocampus (Figure 8.2). The main function of the entorhinal cortex is that of the **olfactory association area**, which allows us to distinguish between different smells. Thus one major input to the entorhinal cortex is from the **olfactory bulb** (cranial nerve I, the nerve of smell). However, it also receives input from many sensory cortical association areas, i.e. those areas that identify and integrate sensory impulses of all kinds entering the brain, a process necessary in order to make sense of the world. This information is channelled through the entorhinal cortex, where some

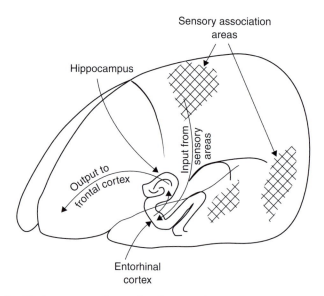

FIGURE 8.3 The hippocampal complex shown within the brain (left side shown) with inputs from the sensory association areas and output to the prefrontal area.

integration may take place. It is then passed on to the hippocampus, enabling it to carry out the major function of influencing thinking via pathways to the prefrontal cortex. The entorhinal cortex appears to be a vital link in the chain of events that leads from the arrival of sensory impulses in the brain to the development of a thought or idea, the *cortical sensory association areas* → *entorhinal cortex* → *hippocampus* → *prefrontal cortex* pathway (Figure 8.3). Clearly, much of our thinking is centred round our responses to sensory stimuli.

The entorhinal cortex is normally composed of six distinct cell layers, like the remaining cerebral cortex but unlike the hippocampus which has three cell layers. In schizophrenia, however, the entorhinal cortex, in particular, shows a loss of **layer ii cells** (Figure 8.2) and abnormal changes in the cytoarchitecture of the remaining cells of layer ii. This kind of structural cellular disruption can only occur during the embryological development of the brain, not later, and therefore the individual is born with these cellular malformations already in place. How this might happen is discussed in the next section. It might be expected that if the individual is born with a brain defect, the symptoms of malfunction will be present from birth. However, the age of onset of symptoms in schizophrenia is usually in the late teens or early twenties, apparently caused by a catastrophic loss of neurons at that time (Thompson *et al.* 2001; Carlson 2001). The question is, however, whether there are any signs during childhood. Some interesting studies have provided evidence that some of those who develop schizophrenia later in life show disturbed patterns of behaviour as a young children (Yakeley and Murray 1996; Roberts *et al.* 1993). The work involved researchers studying old home movies of children at play, watching for disturbances in the children's behaviour, but not knowing which of the children were destined to become schizophrenic. On the basis of the behaviour patterns displayed, researchers picked out those they thought would be prone to schizophrenia, and these were indeed the same children who had developed the disease. This research suggests a preschizophrenic child behaviour pattern, lending weight to the notion that schizophrenia is a neurodevelopmental disorder. The child who is likely to develop schizophrenia later in life has poor abilities to mix and socialise with friends and is likely to underachieve at school (Carlson 2001). It would appear that in **preschizophrenia** the preference for social isolation which is a major negative symptom of the fully developed disease is present to a lesser degree, while attention and language problems are more frequent.

The hippocampus is an important area for memory, and schizophrenic patients often perform poorly on memory-related tasks, further supporting the theory of a disruption in the hippocampal → prefrontal cortex integration (Fletcher 1998). A disruption is also indicated by a **hypofrontality** found in schizophrenic patients, i.e. a reduction in frontal lobe activity during thinking and task-related functions, in its turn indicated by a reduction in the level of **phosphomonoesters** (**PMEs**) in the frontal lobe. PMEs are precursors of phospholipids, the molecular component of cell membranes. **Phosphodiesters** (**PDEs**) are the breakdown products of phospholipids. A change in the PME/PDE ratio, showing a reduction in PME and higher PDE, is an indication of neuronal breakdown and losses and is seen in both dementia and schizophrenia. In fact, PME reduction correlates well with negative symptoms: the lower the PME, the more profound the negative symptoms in schizophrenia (Maier 1999).

The positive symptoms are also intensively investigated, particularly hallucinations. Visual hallucinations may be due to a **disinhibition** effect caused by a reduction in the sensory input to the cortex. This allows the cortex to generate and release its own false *endogenous* sensory stimuli which are then interpreted by the visual cortex as real visual stimuli. It is thought that the normal input of stimuli may have an *inhibitory* effect on the cortex, preventing any such false signals from being produced. An alternative view is that of **cerebral irritation**, such that abnormally high cerebral excitation of the visual memory banks generates the false image (David and Busatto 1999). Given the integrating role of the entorhinal cortex and the hippocampus over a wide range of sensory stimuli, and the disruption of the cells in these areas in schizophrenia, it should not be difficult to see a situation where genuine external sensory stimuli are distorted by the brain.

Auditory hallucinations appear to be the result of left temporal lobe dysfunction. The temporal lobes have the sensory area for hearing (auditory area, Brodmann 41 and 42), and the left temporal lobe in particular specialises in language and speech. Clearly, memory is involved in hallucinations, as indicated by the highly personal nature of most hallucinatory experiences, and therefore the hippocampus must be involved in the aetiology.

The involvement of the left temporal lobe in auditory hallucinations is consistent with the fact that the left hemisphere of the brain has most of the pathology in this disease. This has been termed a **lateralisation**, where one side of the brain is more dominant than the other in the cause of the symptoms (David and Busatto 1999). However, pathology has also been demonstrated in the right hemisphere, although to a lesser extent. Hence schizophrenia is a disorder that is predominantly, but not exclusively, of the left side of the brain. The reason for lateralisation is probably tied up with the way the brain is put together during fetal life, its neurodevelopment.

Neurodevelopment as a factor

The findings that the entorhinal cortex layer ii cell disruption is involved in the symptoms of schizophrenia are consistent with the theories related to the cause of thought disorder and hallucinations. Layer ii cell disruption of the entorhinal cortex could only have happened during the development of the brain in embryo. The central nervous system begins as a tube of cells surrounding a central lumen, formed by the third week of gestation. The lumen is destined to become the brain's ventricular system, filled with cerebrospinal fluid (CSF). At the rostral (*head* end) of the tube, cells (which will become neurons) nearest the lumen are dividing rapidly into many millions from weeks 10 to 22 of gestation. Most of this mitotic division takes place within the **ventricular zone** (**VZ**) nearest to the lumen (Figure 8.4). The next layer out from the VZ is the **subventricular zone** (**SZ**); outside that is the **intermediate zone** (**IZ**); and the outer layer of the tube is the **marginal zone** (**MZ**). The cells of the VZ are anchored by their processes to the lumen on one side and to the SZ on the other side. Each **cell cycle** involves the cell body moving along these processes, undergoing DNA replication (the **S phase** of **interphase**) as it approaches the SZ, and going through **mitosis** when it is close to the lumen. Each cell repeats this cyclic event some 34 or 35 times, resulting in many millions of cells. All these cells must go somewhere, as they cannot all continue to occupy the VZ. Three major waves of cellular migration occur from the VZ outwards to various points beyond the SZ and IZ into the MZ. The first wave involves huge numbers of cells moving to a position just beyond the IZ in the MZ layer. The second wave follows a similar movement, bypassing the first cells and stopping at a point just outside the first cells, i.e. closer to the tube surface. The third wave of migration does the same again, but these cells take up position closer still to the tube surface. Each successive wave of cellular movement, therefore, goes a little further than the previous migration towards the tube surface. Their final position is critical, since once in place the cells cannot return or try another path. If the cells migrate to the wrong position, they will be unable to make the correct synaptic connections and that would disrupt brain function. The process of neuronal migration takes about three months overall and takes place within the **second trimester** of pregnancy; the first wave is complete within 24 hours, but the successive waves take longer as the cortex thickens with cells.

To aid them in the task of correctly finding their way during a migration, neurons rely on specialised glial cells, **radial glia**, to form a frame along which they can travel, like climbing plants growing up a trellis. Once the neuronal migration is complete, the glial cell framework breaks down and disappears. This is one reason why neurons get only one attempt at migration. Other major controlling factors are the chemicals within that part of

NEURAL TUBE

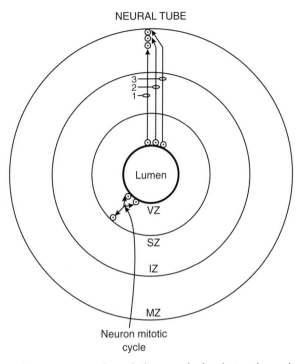

FIGURE 8.4 Schematic section through the neural tube during the early development of the nervous system. VZ is the ventricular zone near the tube lumen. The other zones are SZ (subventricular zone), IZ (intermediate zone) and MZ (marginal zone). Cell mitosis (division) takes place in the VZ, with the cell alternating from close to the lumen (where it divides) to close to the SZ. At specific times, three waves of cell migration out of the VZ into the MZ take place (labelled 1, 2 and 3). The first migration places cells short of the outer layer, but successive migrations place cells closer to the surface.

the primitive brain, many of which are just being discovered. These chemicals are vital, not only for migration but for the post-migrational development of synaptic connections. Neurons are now fixed in their new position for life. From here they must make synaptic connections, perhaps in some cases up to one hundred thousand per neuron, to the other relevant brain areas. They begin the task of growing dendrites and axons, guided by the biochemistry, and these extend to form synaptic connections, i.e. they 'wire-up' the brain. It would appear that in schizophrenia, for reasons still unknown, neurons of several parts of the brain, and layer cells of the entorhinal cortex and cells of the hippocampus in particular, take the wrong route during migration and end up in the wrong place (therefore making wrong synaptic connections) or die (causing neuronal losses). The result is to cause disruption of the functions of the *cortical sensory association areas → entorhinal cortex → hippocampus → prefrontal cortex* pathway (Figure 8.3). The malfunction of this pathway may be the cause of the thought disorder associated with schizophrenia; the hippocampus is unable to make its normal vital input into thought conception, which is therefore distorted and disrupted.

It is interesting that the migration of neuronal cells is accompanied at the same time by a similar migration of cells destined to become skin. It is these cells that form the skin patterns we recognise as fingerprints. Perhaps the disturbance of neuronal migration in the preschizophrenic brain is mirrored by similar disturbances in skin cell migration. Twins were used to investigate this idea, so that their finger and palm prints could be compared. In those pairs of twins in which both twins developed schizophrenia, they had identical skin patterns. However, where only one twin of the pair developed the disease, each twin had a different skin pattern. It now appears that amongst monozygotic (identical) twins the 48% risk of one twin developing schizophrenia if the other already has the disease is only an average figure. A closer look at these twins has identified a range of risks from 10.7% for monozygotic twins who had their own separate placentas (**dichorionic**) to 60% for monozygotic twins who shared the same placenta (**monochorionic**). This last group of twins had not only identical genes but also a virtually identical uterine environment, including the same products delivered through a common placenta. This is powerful evidence for gene and environmental interaction in the causation of schizophrenia.

The biochemical changes in schizophrenia

For many years now it has been recognised that dopamine is, in some way, involved in the production of some of the symptoms of schizophrenia. The *dopamine hypothesis* of schizophrenia was based on observations that drugs like cocaine and the amphetamines caused schizophrenic-like psychotic events, with hallucinations and bizarre behaviour; these drugs were known to increase dopamine levels in the brain. In addition, it was noticed that the **phenothiazine** drugs, some of which were first used as anti-emetics, reduced psychotic symptoms in schizophrenic patients. Since these drugs block the dopamine receptors, it was postulated that excess dopaminergic transmission was the cause of the psychotic symptoms (especially involving the D_2, and possibly the D_3, receptors).

See page 120

Dopamine is the neurotransmitter within four major pathways of the brain (Figure 8.5) (Blows 2000):

1 the **mesocortical tract**, passing from the brain stem to the cerebral cortex (possibly involved in schizophrenia);
2 the **mesolimbic tract**, passing from the brain stem to the limbic system, (the system most likely to be involved in schizophrenia);
3 the **tuberoinfundibular tract**, passing between several nuclei within the hypothalamus and the pituitary stalk (not thought to be involved in schizophrenia);
4 the **nigrostriatal tract**, passing from the substantia nigra (midbrain) to the corpus striatum (basal ganglia) (produces and uses the largest amount of dopamine in the brain, but appears not to be involved in schizophrenia, except in the side-effects of the drugs used to treat the disorder).

The mesolimbic system, thought to be the pathway most involved in positive symptoms, originates in the brain stem (the **ventral tegmental area** of

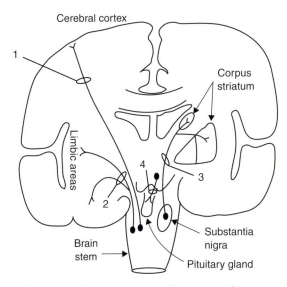

FIGURE 8.5 The four main dopaminergic pathways: (1) the mesocortical pathway (brain stem to cortex); (2) the mesolimbic pathway (brain stem to limbic system); (3) the nigrostriatal pathway (substantia nigra to corpus striatum); (4) the tuberoinfundibular pathway (hypothalamus to pituitary stalk).

the midbrain) and terminates in the limbic system (the **nucleus accumbens** and the **amygdala**; Blows 2000; Wild and Benzel 1994). This pathway and the mesocortical pathway normally use less dopamine than the other dopaminergic tracts, but can sometimes produce excess dopamine. The nucleus accumbens has D_4 receptors, but is especially rich in D_3 receptors, and both receptor types have been found to be raised in some schizophrenics who were drug-free prior to measurement (Carlson 2001). In fact, various studies of dopamine and dopamine receptor levels patients with schizophrenia have proved to be somewhat ambiguous, with relatively normal levels found in some patients (Roberts *et al.* 1993), but disturbed levels found in other patients (Carlson 2001). One way of measuring dopamine levels is to measure the level of the dopamine metabolite called **homovanillic acid** (**HVA**, the waste product of dopamine) excreted via the cerebrospinal fluid (CSF). HVA has been found to be raised in schizophrenic patients, indicating a higher than normal rate of dopamine turnover, and in post-mortem studies has been found localised to the mesocortical and mesolimbic pathways.

The dopamine hypothesis is a neat concept but it has its difficulties, indicating that a more complex picture exists. Although excessive dopamine stimulation of D_2, D_3 and possibly D_4 receptors may be the cause of *some* symptoms, especially the positive symptoms, it is clear that dopamine disturbance is not the *cause* of the disease. There has to be, for example, a cause for the disturbed dopamine levels. This is further illustrated by the fact that the phenothiazine drugs do not cure schizophrenia; patients must usually continue on medication for life, otherwise the symptoms return. Unlike the psychoses seen in cocaine or amphetamine use, the symptoms of schizophrenia are not simply the result of dopamine excess but are part of a much wider pathology. The dopamine hypothesis, therefore, has lost ground as a main cause of the psychoses, and is now seen as just one more small piece of a much larger jigsaw. Other neurotransmitters are involved in this disorder, in particular **glutamate** and **cholecystokinin**, both of which are active in layer ii of the See page 165 entorhinal cortex and are thought to have an important part to play in brain cortical development. Both glutamate and cholecystokinin neurons seem to have a direct dopaminergic innervation in the human brain, suggesting that dopamine disturbance could have a knock-on effect on glutamate and cholecystokinin levels.

The possible role of environmental factors

See page 159 We saw that schizophrenia is considered to be polygenic in origin and, if this is so, it should be possible to identify some environmental factors at work in its aetiology. In fact, while epidemiological studies have suggested some interesting possibilities, modern genetic research is indicating that genes play a much greater role than does any environmental factor. However, two particular environmental factors stand out as significant: a history of birth trauma and maternal influenza during pregnancy.

Schizophrenia shows a higher incidence in those who have a history of cerebral birth trauma, such as prolonged periods of cerebral hypoxia during labour, or who have mothers who had problems during pregnancy, such as pre-eclampsia. Preterm infants subjected to perinatal trauma have a tendency to acquire enlarged ventricles (as seen in schizophrenic patients), identified by brain scanning after birth. There is a link between perinatal complications and neurological abnormalities, and male infants seem to be more prone to lateral ventricular enlargement than female infants as a result of obstetric trauma. The reason is unknown; perhaps it is linked to differences See page 7 in the male and female brains making the male brain more vulnerable. Such trauma may also permanently change some neural connections within the brain which do not show symptoms until maturity.

There is also generally an increased number of infants destined to develop schizophrenia who were born during the late winter and early spring, a period during which viruses are particularly active (e.g. colds and influenza). This may have something to do with a lack of **ultraviolet (UV) light** and **vitamin D** during a winter pregnancy (Furlow 2001). The majority of schizophrenic patients have their birthday in February or March, and the fewest have their birthday in August or September. This has led to speculation that perhaps a virus of some kind has triggered the onset of schizophrenia in a brain previously altered by abnormal neuronal migrations. There is some evidence to suggest that maternal exposure to the influenza virus during the third trimester of pregnancy increases the risk of schizophrenia in the infant. The role of the virus in this disease is the subject of much debate and research. A possible mechanism is that antibodies created in the maternal blood designed to destroy the virus may cross the placenta into the fetal circulation, enter the offspring's brain and interfere with neuronal development. Alternatively, the virus itself may enter the fetal blood and thus the

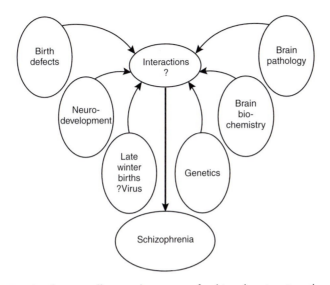

Figure 8.6 The factors affecting the cause of schizophrenia. Somehow they all contribute towards the disease, but their exact interactions, leading to the disease, are unknown.

fetal nervous system. If the virus caused the damage soon after birth, then one interesting suggestion is that such a virus could have entered the brain via the trigeminal nerve (cranial nerve V) (Torrey 1991). If this nerve is followed backwards from the mouth (the site of entry of many viruses, notably colds and influenza), it is seen to enter the brain stem not far from the temporal lobe and the entorhinal cortex. It is also known that some viruses are prone to tract along nerves, as seen in the disease shingles. If this is a possibility, the viral infection could be one more insult in a chain of neurological insults that starts with some abnormal genes and ends with the fully developed disease.

However, this chain of events is far from clear. The problem facing neurobiologists now is piecing the pieces of the jigsaw together (Figure 8.6). It is not known how the genes and environmental factors interact, or how they in turn affect the embryonic neuronal migration, or how this disturbs the biochemistry, or how these all together cause symptoms. There is much still to learn, but we have come a long way since the 1960s when hardly any of the possibilities described above were known. With the advances being made in both neurobiology and understanding of the human genome, the prospects of solving this particular jigsaw puzzle are better now than they ever were.

The antipsychotic drugs

Drugs are used to control the symptoms of schizophrenia and thereby improve the quality of life for the patient, but schizophrenia as a disease remains incurable. The antipsychotic drugs fall into several groups: the phenothiazines (which are further divided into three subgroups), the atypical

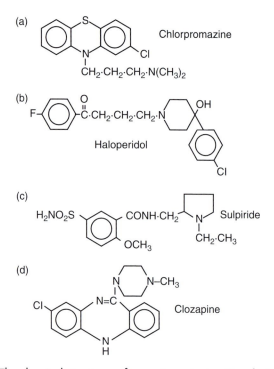

FIGURE 8.7 The chemical structures of some important antipsychotic drugs.

antipsychotics, the butyrophenones, the diphenylbutylpiperidines, the thioxanthenes and the substituted benzamides. The main effects of these drugs are to reduce the positive symptoms of psychosis, to calm the effects of bizarre behaviour and to improve the patient's ability to interact more with their environment.

Phenothiazines

Of these drugs the most commonly used are the phenothiazines. One of their early uses was as anti-emetics, but it was soon recognised that in schizo-phrenic patients they also resulted in a reduction of positive symptoms. A principal member of this drug group is **chlorpromazine** (**Largactil**), which has been said by some to have played a key role in enabling the closure of the big Victorian psychiatric hospitals in favour of community care.

Chlorpromazine (Figure 8.7a) and the other phenothiazines are dopamine receptor **antagonists**; that is, they bind to and block the dopamine receptor sites, preventing dopamine from binding and having its effect. This dopamine blockade has for years been thought to be the mechanism of symptom pre-vention, lending further support to the dopamine hypothesis. However, this is not the full story of the activity of these drugs. Blocking of the dopamine receptors also has the effect of increasing the metabolism of dopamine, i.e. altering the production and destruction of dopamine, as noted by a measur-able increase in dopamine metabolites (or waste products). This may have

TABLE 8.4 The effects and side-effects of the phenothiazine antipsychotic drugs

Drug	Desired effect	Side-effects
Aliphatics		
Chlorpromazine	Strong sedation, antipsychotic	Extrapyramidal, hypotension, hypothermia
Methotrimeprazine		
Piperidines		
Thioridazine	Moderate sedation, antipsychotic	Few extrapyramidal
Pipothiazine		
Piperazines		
Fluphenazine	Weak sedation, variable anti-emetic, antipsychotic	Pronounced extrapyramidal
Trifluoperazine		
Perphenazine		
Prochlorperazine		

a longer-term effect on the brain chemistry of the patient, an effect that persists beyond the duration of the drug's activity, including prolonged changes to dopamine receptor activity and sensitivity. Chlorpromazine and the other phenothiazines are tricyclic (three-ringed) compounds (Figure 8.7a), with two outer carbon rings and a central pyridine ring. Each member of this group of drugs has different side branches in place of the chlorine (Cl) and the $CH_2.CH_2.CH_2.N(CH_3)_2$ chain found in chlorpromazine. Three sub-groups of phenothiazine are recognised: the **aliphatics** (e.g. chlorpromazine and methotrimeprazine), the **piperidines** (e.g. thioridazine, pipothiazine) and the **piperazines** (e.g. prochlorperazine, trifluoperazine, perphenazine and fluphenazine). The inclusion of prochlorperazine (Stemetil) in this last group is a measure of the continuing importance of some of these drugs as anti-emetics as well as antipsychotics. In terms of sedatory effects (i.e. calming the patient without any loss of consciousness), the aliphatics are the most potent and the piperazines are the weakest. The main effects and side-effects of the phenothiazine drugs are listed in Table 8.4.

As dopamine antagonists, the phenothiazine drugs prevent the direct effect of dopamine on its receptors within the four main dopamine pathways of the brain. In schizophrenia, the most important pathway in which to See page 44 block dopamine is thought to be the *mesolimbic* tract, but the activity of these drugs is not exclusive to this tract. They block dopamine receptors also in the other tracts, and such a blockade results in side-effects, notably the extrapyramidal symptoms known as **parkinsonism** (tremor, stiffness of limbs and walking difficulties), **dystonia** (abnormal movements of the face and body), **akathisia** (motor system restlessness) and late onset **tardive dyskinesia** (abnormal repeated oral and facial movements such as lip sucking or smacking, lateral jaw movements and flicking of the tongue, which may be irreversible). These are associated with dopamine blockade

See page 224

of the *nigrostriatal* pathway within the basal ganglia (Blows 2000). Parkinsonism is so named because it resembles Parkinson's disease but, unlike the disease, parkinsonism is reversible by reducing or changing the medication, or by adding anti-Parkinson drugs to the prescription. Other side-effects include **hypotension** (low blood pressure), due to a depressive effect on the **vasomotor centres** of the brain stem that regulate blood pressure, and **hypothermia** (low body temperature), especially in the elderly, due to the drugs' activity on the temperature control centre within the **hypothalamus**. Some of these drugs, such as chlorpromazine, can interfere with the balance of some hormones, causing increased **prolactin** production (which can stimulate breast milk production in either sex), decreased **growth hormone** and **gonadotrophins** (those hormones affecting the ovaries or testes), and variations in the levels of **adrenocorticotropic hormone (ACTH)** released, depending on the drug dosage. ACTH regulates the release of cortisol from the adrenal cortex, a hormone particularly

See page 140

important in stress.

Butyrophenones

See page 145

Drugs more specific to one of the subtypes of dopamine receptor, especially D_2, would be more efficient, with fewer side-effects for the patient than the phenothiazines. A selective D_2 receptor inhibitor would, at least, avoid the complications of blocking the other receptors (especially D_1) (Blows 2000) as the phenothiazines appear to do. Such a drug is **haloperidol** (Figure 8.7b), a member of another group, the butyrophenones, which also includes **benperidol** and **droperidol**. These are all potent antipsychotics with few sedative properties, but they can produce extrapyramidal side-effects by D_2 blockade in the nigrostriatal pathway. They have a different chemical structure from the phenothiazines, in that they are not tricyclic (see haloperidol structure, Figure 8.7b). Haloperidol has a one hundred times greater affinity for the D_2 receptor than for the D_1 receptor and is therefore a more selective D_2 receptor antagonist than any of the phenothiazines. As a potent antipsychotic, haloperidol is very useful as a treatment for acute psychotic states as it causes a quick recovery of normal behaviour.

Thioxanthenes

The thioxanthenes group contains two main drugs: **flupenthixol**, which is useful in the treatment of withdrawn and apathetic patients, and **zuclopenthixol**, which should not be used in patients with predominantly negative symptoms but is a suitable treatment for agitation and aggression in schizophrenia.

Diphenylbutylpiperidines

The diphenylbutylpiperidines, of which the main member is **pimozide**, are similar in action to the butyrophenones, being potent antipsychotics, but with extrapyramidal and potential cardiac side-effects.

Substituted benzamides

The substituted benzamides includes the drug **sulpiride** (Figure 8.7c), which can control severe positive symptoms when given in high dosage or improve activity in those affected by dominant negative symptoms if given in lower dose. Sulpiride appears to have a greater affinity for the D_2 receptor than for any of the other dopamine receptors.

Atypicals

The newer atypical antipsychotics include the drugs **clozapine** (Figure 8.7d), which is used for schizophrenic patients who do not respond to other drug treatments, as well as **risperidone**, **olanzapine**, **quetiapine** and **amisulpride**. These drugs produce fewer extrapyramidal symptoms, possibly because they are more specific to the *mesocortical tract* dopamine receptors. They also See page 44 cause less prolactin disturbance than the older phenothiazine drugs, but clozapine can cause blood **dyscrasia** (serious disturbance of the number of blood cells in circulation, sometimes causing dangerous falls in the leucocyte count). As a result, patients treated with this drug must be in hospital and registered on a special monitoring service.

Clozapine metabolites have been found to inhibit the growth of the **human immunodeficiency virus** (**HIV**, the known cause of **acquired immunodeficiency syndrome**, **AIDS**) and, while HIV is not known to be involved in schizophrenia, this discovery has added weight to the theory that an unknown virus may be involved in the cause (see environmental factors). See page 172 Perhaps other antipsychotic drugs, or their metabolites, work by a similar viral blocking action in the long term, and studies involving the treatment of schizophrenic patients with known antiviral drugs are now under way. Apart from being a dopamine receptor antagonist, clozapine has other properties; notably it is a potent sedative and also a serotonin receptor antagonist. Also, unlike the phenothiazines, which bind mainly to the D_1 and D_2 receptors, clozapine has an almost equal affinity for both the D_2 and D_3 receptors, and the inclusion of D_3 receptors in this drug's activity may be a key in the further understanding of the importance of the dopamine hypothesis in this disease. It is possible that there is a higher number of D_3 See page 170 receptors than any of the others within the limbic system, i.e. the *mesolimbic* pathway. See page 44

Drug therapy has become the main mechanism in the management of patients' symptoms. However, one problem with drug therapy in schizophrenia is that of poor patient compliance, particularly within the community. Failure to take the drugs regularly results in the repeated return of some patients to hospital. To improve patient compliance, some drugs such as fluphenazine are available as **depot** injections, i.e. oil-based slow-releasing intramuscular medication that can be given by the nurse. This is one of several ways in which nurses can improve patient compliance with their medication regime (Coffey 1999).

The overall picture of the biology of schizophrenia is very difficult to put together. There are hundreds of factors involved, many of them beyond our current understanding. The five main classes of factors are genetic, environmental, neurodevelopmental, biochemical and pathological. Much work is in progress in an effort to pull these separate threads together, to see how they interact, and to produce an integrated understanding of the aetiology of the disease. This chapter has outlined the position so far, but much more is to come. No 'cure' or effective prevention of schizophrenia is likely until the complete picture is in place.

Key points

- Schizophrenia is a neurodevelopmental disorder.
- The symptoms of schizophrenia fall into two categories, positive and negative.
- The risk of developing schizophrenia is about 1% for the population as a whole.
- The disease is probably polygenic (several genes involved interacting with environmental factors).
- Some abnormalities have been reported in the brain. These include enlarged ventricles, a reduction in brain weight of about 5% and a shortening of the length of the brain.
- The entorhinal cortex and the anterior hippocampus both show neuron losses of about 20%, and a change in the cytoarchitecture.
- The entorhinal cortex appears to be a vital link between the sensory areas of the brain to the prefrontal cortex, i.e. the *cortical sensory association areas → entorhinal cortex → hippocampus → prefrontal cortex* pathway.
- The entorhinal cortex shows a neuronal loss and abnormal cytoarchitecture of layer ii cells.
- Preschizophrenia, the presymptom childhood stages, causes the child to have poor abilities to mix and socialise with friends, with attention and language problems causing them to underachieve at school.
- Visual hallucinations may be due to a disinhibition or a cerebral irritation effect. Auditory hallucinations may involve abnormal left temporal lobe activity.
- Although both cerebral hemispheres are involved, schizophrenia shows some degree of lateralisation, where the left side of the brain has more dominant pathology than the right side.
- Schizophrenia also shows a hypofrontality, i.e. a reduction in frontal lobe activity, indicated by lower levels of phosphomonoesters (PMEs).
- The mesolimbic system is thought to be the pathway most involved in positive symptoms. It originates in the brain stem (the ventral tegmental area) and terminates in the limbic system (the nucleus accumbens and the amygdala).
- The dopamine hypothesis of schizophrenia was based on observations that drugs like cocaine and the amphetamines cause schizophrenic-like psychotic events because these drugs increase dopamine levels in the brain.
- Homovanillic acid (HVA, the waste product of dopamine) is excreted via the cerebrospinal fluid (CSF), and is raised in many living schizophrenic

patients, indicating a higher than normal rate of dopamine turnover. Dopamine has been localised to the mesocortical and mesolimbic pathways.

- Glutamate and cholecystokinin, both of which are active in layer ii of the entorhinal cortex, may be involved in the biochemistry of schizophrenia.
- Two factors stand out as significant environmental contributors to the cause of schizophrenia: a history of birth trauma and maternal influenza during pregnancy.
- The antipsychotic drugs fall into several groups: the phenothiazines (which are further divided into three subgroups), the atypical antipsychotics, the butyrophenones, the diphenylbutylpiperidines, the thioxanthenes and the substituted benzamides.
- As dopamine antagonists, the phenothiazine drugs prevent the direct effect of dopamine on its receptors.
- In schizophrenia, the most important pathway in which to block dopamine is thought to be the *mesolimbic* tract, but phenothiazines also block dopamine receptors in other tracts resulting in extrapyramidal side-effects known as parkinsonism.

References

Blows W. (2000) Neurotransmitters of the brain: serotonin, noradrenaline (norepinephrine), and dopamine. *Journal of Neuroscience Nursing*, **32** (4): 234–238.

Carlson N. R. (2001) *Physiology of Behavior* (7th edn). Allyn and Bacon, Boston.

Coffey M. (1999) Psychosis and medication: strategies for improving adherence. *British Journal of Nursing*, **8** (4): 225–230.

David A. S. and Busatto G. (1999) The hallucination: a disorder of brain and mind, *in* Ron M. A. and David A. S. (eds), *Disorders of Brain and Mind*. Cambridge University Press, Cambridge.

Fletcher P. (1998) The missing link: a failure of fronto-hippocampal integration in schizophrenia. *Nature Neuroscience*, **1** (4): 266–267.

Furlow B. (2001) The making of a mind. *New Scientist*, **171** (2300): 38–41.

Holland M., Baguley I. and Davies T. (1999) Psychological methods of treating hallucinations and delusions: 1. *British Journal of Nursing*, **8** (15): 998–1002.

Maier M. (1999) Magnetic resonance spectroscopy in neuropsychiatry, *in* Ron M. A. and David A. S. (eds), *Disorders of Brain and Mind*. Cambridge University Press, Cambridge.

Roberts G. W., Leigh P. N. and Weinberger D. R. (1993) *Neuropsychiatric Disorders*. Wolfe, London.

Taylor E. (1999) Early disorders and later schizophrenia, *in* Ron M. A. and David A. S. (eds), *Disorders of Brain and Mind*. Cambridge University Press, Cambridge.

Thompson P. M., Vidal C., Giedd J. N., Gochman P., Blumenthal J., Nicolson R., Toga A. W. and Rapoport J. L. (2001) Mapping adolescent brain change reveals dynamic wave of accelerated gray matter loss in very early-onset schizophrenia. *Proceedings of the National Academy of Sciences of the USA*, **98** (20): 11650–11655.

Torrey E. F. (1991) A viral-anatomical explanation of schizophrenia. *Schizophrenia Bulletin*, **17** (1): 15–18.

Wild G. C. and Benzel E. C. (1994) *Essential of Neurochemistry*. Jones and Bartlett, Boston.

Yakeley J. W. and Murray R. M. (1996) Schizophrenia. *Medicine*, **24** (2): 6–10.

Chapter 9

Depression

- Introduction
- Factors in the aetiology of depression
- Brain pathology
- Biochemistry and immunity in depression
- Post-partum depression and Seasonal Affective Disorder (SAD)
- The antidepressant drugs
- Mood-stabilising drugs
- Key points

Introduction

It is not unnatural to be unhappy as a result of certain life events, such as bereavement of a close family member, and this kind of reaction is expected. It is also expected that the depressive state will resolve itself after a reasonable period of time, allowing the individual concerned to return to their usual state of mind and to function normally. Depressive illness occurs either when the depressed state has no apparent cause or reason or when the period of depression is prolonged beyond what is considered normal, with no signs of recovery. The depth of depression is important also. A depressive illness dominates the person's life, committing them to an existence in misery with no end in sight. Suicide becomes an attractive way out of this despair and many depressive patients succeed in killing themselves to end their suffering. Such patients need help to recover the purpose of living and, with treatment, many are returned successfully to a happier existence. Such an outcome is more likely now than it has ever been as a result of better

TABLE 9.1 Previous and current classifications of depression

Previous classifications	Explanation
1. Primary	Not associated with any other disorder
Secondary	As a result of some other disorder
2. Neurotic	Mild depression, associated with symptoms of a nervous nature, like anxiety
Psychotic	More severe depression, associated with psychotic symptoms akin to schizophrenia
3. Reactive	Caused by a sad or unfortunate life event, and continued from there
Endogenous	From within, i.e. no identifiable life event is recognised as the cause
Current classification	
Unipolar	Depressive symptoms only
Bipolar	Depressive symptoms plus bouts of mania

understanding of what is happening in the brains of depressed patients and of the introduction of improved drug treatment.

Various attempts have been made in the past to classify different depressed states and some of these classifications have been adopted and used more commonly than others (Table 9.1). The current view is that there are two main types of depressive illness, **unipolar depression** (having symptoms of depression only) and **bipolar depression** (having symptoms of depression coupled with periods of mania). This view is supported by growing evidence concerning the underlying biology of depression (Carlson 2001). Depressed patients demonstrate the symptoms we now associate with disturbed receptor and neurotransmitter levels in the brain (Table 9.2).

Another disorder, in which depressive symptoms appear to be chronic and directed *outwards* towards the world in the form of anger or irritability, is called **dysthymic disorder**.

See page 188

Factors in the aetiology of depression

The cause of depression is basically unknown. Genes have been implicated for many years because some forms of depression appear to be familial, particularly the more severe manic-depressive bipolar disorder. For the population as a whole, the risk of developing unipolar depression is 6%, and for bipolar depression the risk is 1% (the same as for schizophrenia). Mild forms of depression carry a general population risk of approximately 10%. The first-degree relatives of a patient with bipolar depression have a concordance rate of 19% – i.e. a 19% chance of developing the disease – while for unipolar depression the concordance rate is 10%. The concordance rate for bipolar depression in monozygotic (identical) twins is about 65%, and in dizygotic (fraternal) twins the concordance rate is about 14%. Affected twins are most likely to have the same disorder, i.e. if one has the bipolar form then the other will have the bipolar form, although occasional crossing

TABLE 9.2 The symptoms of depression

Symptom	Further explanation
Low level of mood (flattening of affect)	Misery which does not improve; looks very unhappy
Pessimistic thoughts	Feelings of hopelessness, unworthiness, no self-confidence
Low energy	
Psychomotor retardation	Slow body movements, delayed responses to stimuli
Sleep disturbance and tiredness	Early morning waking
Poor appetite and weight loss	
Slow speech and thought	Protracted conversations
Loss of libido	
Sometimes anxiety, agitation or restlessness	
Severe depression is sometimes associated with loss of reality and pessimistic delusions	These symptoms are akin to those of schizophrenia. Delusions are of doom and gloom
Sometimes mania (in bipolar depression)	Mania is the sudden outburst of overactivity, rapid speech and thinking, expanded optimistic ideas, increased appetite and libido, possibly aggression and psychotic symptoms like hallucinations. Manic events occur between depressive periods but are rare compared to the depressive phases

over has been seen. All these figures are much greater than for the population as a whole, suggesting a powerful genetic influence in the causation of this disorder.

The genes themselves have not been found, although certain genes on chromosomes 11, 18, 21 and X have attracted interest. Of these, a gene on chromosome 11 has not proved significant, but an X-linked form of bipolar disorder has been located to Xq28 (**major affective disorder 2**, or *MAFD2*), accounting for a subset of familial bipolar patients, possibly about one-third of the total number of sufferers. The reader may recognise this genetic locus as the site for several other disorders involving mental retardation which are *See page 90* identified in this book (see Table 5.2, and Rett syndrome). The difference between unipolar and bipolar disorder is emphasised by the fact that the incidence for the unipolar form in females is double that seen in males, while in bipolar disorder there is no difference between the sexes.

Bipolar disorder has shown a tendency to develop more often in those persons born in the winter months (not unlike schizophrenia), leading to a suspect viral origin. One proposed virus is **Borna virus**, which is known to infect animals, notably horses. It is responsible for a significant number of horse deaths. Viruses fall mainly into two camps, the **DNA (deoxyribosenucleic acid)** form, and the **RNA (ribosenucleic acid)** form. Borna virus is a single-stranded RNA virus that may find its way from animals to man. Evidence for the presence of Borna virus in depressed patients is growing (Mestel 1997), but this is just one of several suggested environmental factors that are possibly involved in the cause of depression. Other factors include maternal deprivation, unstable parental relationships and disturbance in the home life, all factors resulting in an unhappy childhood. These factors will have led to various *losses*, i.e. loss of a loved one, a job or a home. Sudden loss events, such as a bereavement or parental separation, may trigger the first bouts of depression in a vulnerable individual. In adulthood, people who lost one or both parents before the age of 11 years are particularly vulnerable to depression (Thompson 1996). Environmental factors appear to play a much bigger role in the aetiology of unipolar depression, while genetic factors are more important in bipolar disorder.

Suicide is a phenomenon that is often triggered by environmental factors such as poor social conditions or very difficult personal circumstances, all of which cause chronic stress. Brown (1997) reports that the highest suicide rate in the world is in China, the country with the largest population. China has 22% of the world population but 40% of the world suicides. Here, the victims are mainly women (one in four female deaths between the ages of 15 to 44 years), although everywhere else the male suicide rate is greater than the female rate. Since 1990 some two million Chinese have killed themselves. Other countries are also affected, although to a lesser extent, and Brown (1997) describes *the suicide belt* as being from China to Sri Lanka via Hong Kong and Taiwan (Figure 9.1). Despite the very high rate of suicide it is considered that mental illness, and in particular depression, probably accounts for only about 50% of the Chinese deaths. While

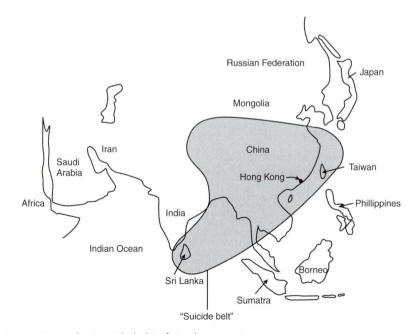

FIGURE 9.1 The 'suicide belt' of South-east Asia.

See page 46 links between brain chemistry and suicide can be established in many cases (see serotonin), it is clear that environmental factors are extremely important.

Brain pathology

The evidence of physical changes identified in the brain during depression is limited. In many cases, the brains of depressed and normal persons, previously examined at post mortem but these days seen on brain scans, are virtually identical. Changes are sometimes observed which are akin to those found in schizophrenia; for example, between 10% and 30% of depressed patients have some degree of ventricular enlargement and some patients show a reduction in the size of the temporal lobe. The frontal and temporal lobes also suffer some cell losses in *elderly* depressed patients, but the extensive loss of cells from the cerebral cortex seen in a significant number of schizophrenic patients has not been found in bipolar depression (Ron 1999). Lesions are sometimes found in the periventricular white matter, i.e. the axons surrounding the ventricles. Studies of cerebral blood flow indicate various changes in the left anterior and right posterior areas of the cerebrum in a number of patients, including reduced blood flow to the left anterior cingulate gyrus and the left dorsolateral prefrontal cortex (Figure 9.2). Ron (1999) suggests that symptoms of mood disorder are most likely to arise in the case of dysfunction of the temporal and frontal lobe cortex (or subcortex), combined with either the temporal lobe associated limbic areas, or the pathway from the basal ganglia to the cortex via the thalamus.

To summarise, the brains of depressed patients show some mild schizophrenic-like changes affecting the function of the frontal and temporal lobes in association with the limbic system.

Biochemistry and immunity in depression

The main changes seen in the brains of depressed patients begin at molecular level. Overall, this is a disease of brain chemistry disturbance, an imbalance between several neurotransmitters and their receptors. The following text should be read in conjunction with Chapter 3.

Serotonin (5-hydroxytryptamine, or 5-HT)

Serotonin is a major neurotransmitter in one of the two **diffuse modulatory systems** extending from the **raphe nuclei** of the brain stem to many See page 186 other brain areas (Figure 9.3a) (Blows 2000a). Serotonin levels have been identified as a factor in depression. The neurotransmitter's metabolites (waste products for excretion), derived from degraded serotonin and measured in the cerebrospinal fluid (CSF), are significantly *reduced* in depression, indicating a lower than average turnover of the transmitter at the synapse. Very low levels of serotonin have been linked to increased violent behaviour, both against the self, as in suicide, or against others, as in violent crime

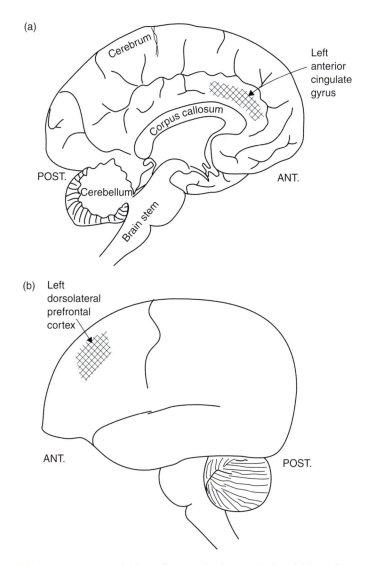

(a)

Cerebrum

Left anterior cingulate gyrus

Corpus callosum

POST.

Cerebellum

Brain stem

ANT.

(b) Left dorsolateral prefrontal cortex

ANT.

POST.

FIGURE 9.2 Depression and blood flow to the brain. Reduced blood flow is often found in (a) the left anterior cingulate gyrus (seen here in midline section of the brain), and (b) the left dorsolateral prefrontal cortex (seen here in a left lateral view of the brain).

including murder (Wild and Benzel 1994; see also aggression). In addition, increases in the numbers of serotonin receptors have been identified in some patients, and this greater receptor density is to be expected if the neurotransmitter is low (Nemeroff 1998). The additional receptors are often of the subtype 2 (i.e. 5-HT2), and this is regarded as a compensatory *up-regulation* of the receptor to maximise the binding of what serotonin there is present. The subtype 2 receptor is thought to be the most important of all the receptor subtypes involved in mood regulation. There is some

See page 148

See page 48

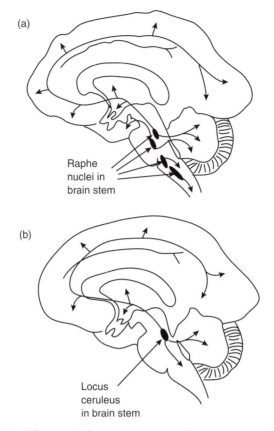

(a)

Raphe
nuclei in
brain stem

(b)

Locus
ceruleus
in brain stem

Figure 9.3 The diffuse modulatory systems. (a) The serotonin pathways from the raphe nuclei in the brain stem extend to many areas of the brain. (b) A similar pattern of noradrenaline pathways extends out from the locus ceruleus of the brain stem.

evidence indicating that the effects of low serotonin are further aggravated by a reduction in serotonin receptor activity (i.e. receptors function less well even when the neurotransmitter binds) and by a loss in the number of neurons within the serotonin pathways, leading to reduced serotonin synthesis.

Serotonin has some effect on the production of noradrenaline in the brain, and lower than normal serotonin levels reduce the noradrenergic neurons' ability to produce noradrenaline. Thus a low serotonin level has a *knock-on* effect in causing a lower noradrenaline level in the brain.

Serotonin also acts on **platelets** (**thrombocytes**), which are blood cells important for the prevention of bleeding by the formation of a **thrombus** (a blood clot). The role of serotonin in relation to platelets is still under investigation, but it seems likely that serotonin enters the platelet and this increases the cell's ability to take in other activating chemical signals. In depression, the platelets show less ability to take up serotonin and thus are less able to be activated.

Noradrenaline

Noradrenaline pathways form the second of the two diffuse modulatory systems in the brain, noradrenaline being centred on the **locus coeruleus** in the brain stem, with pathways to many diverse parts of the cerebral cortex and limbic system (Figure 9.3b) (Blows 2000a). Some evidence indicates disturbance in the numbers and density of noradrenaline receptors in depression (Nemeroff 1998). Of the two major noradrenaline receptors that are known, the increased density appears to be of the beta-adrenergic type. As noted, some serotonin pathways from the raphe nucleus extend to areas that involve noradrenaline secretion, and it seems likely that noradrenaline levels are disturbed because there is a loss of serotonin regulation of noradrenaline secretion.

See page 186

See page 46

Noradrenaline is the neurotransmitter of arousal, i.e. it causes increased levels of brain activity, and it is therefore most active during the day (Blows 2000a).

Dopamine and others

Dopamine is not the major player in the aetiology of depressive symptoms that it is in schizophrenia. Not only is serotonin a regulator of noradrenaline secretion, it also regulates the secretion of dopamine, so disturbance of the serotonin levels seen in depression are likely to have a knock-on effect on dopamine production. It is possible that severe bipolar depressive states that show psychotic symptoms such as hallucinations have some disturbance to the dopaminergic systems, although direct involvement of dopamine in depression has not been demonstrated (Carlson 2001).

The inhibitory role of gamma-aminobutyric acid (GABA) may also be impaired.

Hormones

Hormonal abnormalities are also well recognised in depression. Depressed patients often show reduced levels of secretion of several pituitary hormones, especially growth hormone and thyroid hormone. Depression is frequently associated with **hypothyroidism** and thyroid hormone is given to a number of depressed patients along with their antidepressant medication. Chronic stress, in which persistently high levels of cortisol, and in particular prolonged elevated levels of corticotropin-releasing factor (CRF), can also lead to depression. In this case the **hypathalomo–pituitary–adrenal axis (HPA axis)** (Figure 9.4) goes into prolonged hyperactivity, resulting in enlargement of both the adrenal and pituitary glands. This hyperactivity is probably due to malfunction of the CRF-producing neurons in the hypothalamus and can happen either as a result of external chronic stress or as a result of a direct problem with the neurons. CRF produced in elevated quantities does more than just cause the release of ACTH, it also suppresses sleep (causing **insomnia**), reduces appetite (causing **anorexia**), inhibits reproductive behaviour and causes withdrawal in unfamiliar

See page 65

See page 66

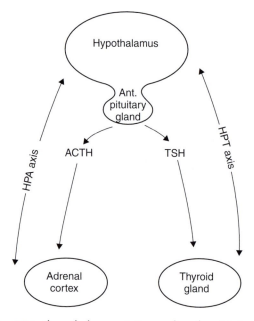

FIGURE 9.4 The HPA (hypothalamo–pituitary–adrenal axis) involves adrenocorticotropic hormone (ACTH). The HPT (hypothalamo–pituitary–thyroid axis) involves thyroid-stimulating hormone (TSH). Depression often involves a prolonged hyperactivity of the HPA, whilst dysthymic disorder involves a dysfunction of the HPT.

environments – all reductions that are seen in depression (Nemeroff 1998). CRF levels are found to be high in the cerebrospinal fluid (CSF) of depressed patients but return to normal with treatment. The increased activity of the HPA axis results in persistently high levels of circulating cortisol, the protective hormone released in stress. Normally, a high level of cortisol in the blood is short-lived, as a result of the hormone binding to receptors in the brain; the brain responds to this by signalling the reduction of cortisol production and release through the HPA axis (Figure 9.5). In depression, these cortisol receptors are not functioning adequately; the brain's ability to suppress cortisol production is reduced and cortisol levels remain high.

In **dysthymic disorder**, there is less evidence for the involvement of the HPA, but there are indications of dysfunction of the **hypathalamo–pituitary–thyroid axis (HPT)** (Figure 9.5) causing thyroid hormones abnormalities in many cases.

Immunity

The relatively new science of **psychoimmunology** is pointing the way towards a better understanding of how the mind (or the brain) affects the immune system and vice versa. Stress and depression are said to be the major players in this field, with significant changes occurring in the immune system in both these disorders. However, the problem of 'cause or effect' comes into play, and much detail has to be worked out to determine whether

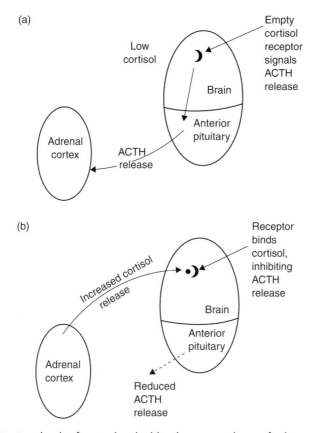

FIGURE 9.5 Low levels of cortisol in the blood cause a release of adrenocorticotropic hormone (ACTH), which stimulates cortisol release from the adrenal cortex (a). This is because cortisol receptors in the brain remain empty and signal the anterior pituitary where ACTH is produced. Increased cortisol in the blood (b) binds with the brain receptors, and this deactivates the signal to the anterior pituitary, which reduces ACTH release. In depression, the receptors are possibly malfunctioning, and ACTH release is not turned off even when cortisol levels are high.

the changes seen cause depression or whether they are the result of depression. Different researchers have reported a wide range of immune changes in depression (Brown 2001), but the main changes are as listed in Table 9.3.

Monocytes are phagocytic white cells; that is, they engulf **antigens** (foreign particles) as part of the fight against infection. **NK (natural killer) cells** are white blood cells that are normally active against virally infected and some malignant cells. **Lymphocytes** are white cells which provide the main defence against invading antigens. There are two types of lymphocytes: **B-cells**, which produce proteins called **antibodies** that attack antigens (B-cell defence is called **humoral immunity**), and **T-cells**, which attack and destroy specific antigens (T-cell defence is called **cell-mediated immunity**). Lymphocyte studies in depression appear conflicting, with overall numbers down but T-cells levels raised. This is possibly because different

TABLE 9.3 The psychoimmunological changes reported in depression

Psychoimmunological change	Possible effects on the patient
Lower circulating active monocytes	?Affects immune response to infection
Lower circulating active NK cells	?May disturb sleep and cause psychomotor retardation
Lower lymphocyte proliferation	?Affects immune response to infection
Increased circulating cytokines	?May be involved in the cause of depression
Raised acute-phase proteins (APP)	?Part of an acute immune response
Raised anti-serotonin antibodies	?Antibodies lower serotonin in blood + CNS
Raised anti-ganglioside antibodies	?Antibodies lower gangliosides in CNS
Raised circulating T-cells	Unknown if any
Disturbed blood lipid levels (HDL)	Unknown if any
Lower circulating beta-endorphin	Associated with lower NK cells
Raised leukocytes, e.g. neutrophils	Unknown if any

subgroups of depressive patients show different lymphocyte results, with overall disturbance affecting cell-mediated immunity more than humoral immunity. Humoral antibody production sometimes involves anti-serotonin antibodies, the presence of which is associated with a poor response to treatment. Understanding these variations is a goal for further research. **Gangliosides** (Table 9.3) are **glycolipids** (i.e. lipids with sugars attached) found in the brain and nervous system. **High-density lipoproteins (HDL)** are blood lipid particles containing **cholesterol**.

Cytokines are chemicals involved in 'cell signalling' during an immune response. Those raised in depression are reported as **interleukin-1beta (IL-1β)**, **interleukin-6 (IL-6)** and **gamma-interferon (γ-IF)**. IL-1β and II-6 appear to be involved in the disturbance of the HPA axis and in the disorder of serotonin metabolism. Brown (2001) reported that patients taking either one of two drugs to boost their immune systems to fight infection or cancer were becoming depressed, and even suicidal. These drugs are **alpha-interferon (α-IF)** and **interleukin-2 (IL-2)**, and it is this kind of observation that provides further weight in support of the **'immune theory'** of depression. The mechanism is still not fully sorted out, but it would appear that cytokines *See page 46* reduce the level of **tryptophan**, the precursor of serotonin, leading to a serotonin shortage. Cytokines are naturally produced during infections by activated immune cells, i.e. leukocytes such as monocytes and lymphocytes. Observations of people with active immune systems during infections show them often to be sad and not eating or sleeping well, symptoms akin to those of depression, and this is sometimes called **'sickness behaviour'**. It may be that depression is, in some cases, a side-effect of inflammatory cytokine activity and that antidepressants may have an anti-inflammatory effect. There is growing evidence that some antidepressant drugs could act as a *prophylaxis*, i.e. have a preventive effect, if given before or during cytokine therapy.

The large circulatory cytokine molecules, such as interleukin, are not generally able to cross the blood–brain barrier, so their role is copied by smaller molecules such as **prostaglandins** and **nitric oxide** *inside* the brain.

These smaller molecules stimulate glial cells in the brain to produce further inflammatory cytokines, which then bind to receptors on neurons of the cerebellum, the hippocampus and the hypothalamus, areas where mood and behaviour are moderated.

As noted, cortisol levels are high in depression, and this has implications for the immune system. Apart from the glial cells of the brain, the immune cells in the blood also have cortisol receptors and can therefore bind cortisol. As well as the HPA axis, inflammatory cytokines also trigger cortisol release, but the rise in cortisol causes the inflammatory cells to reduce cytokine production in a double feedback mechanism (Figure 9.6). If brain cortisol receptors are not working well, inflammatory cell receptors may not be functioning properly either, and the high cortisol levels fail to reduce the cytokine level. A vicious circle is created in which the cytokines continue to stimulate further cortisol release, which is then unable to turn the cytokines off.

See page 188

Some of these findings may also be useful as **markers** of depression since their blood measurement is fairly consistent and they could be used as part of the diagnostic procedure to identify depression. The markers include raised **leucocyte** (white cell) numbers, especially the **neutrophils** (phagocytic cells, of the **granulocyte** white cell group), and the HDL findings.

Whether these immune changes are triggered by a viral infection, as suspected by some, remains to be confirmed. Perhaps depression is of viral origin, or perhaps the effect of depression is to degrade the immune system and to allow viral infections to gain entry.

Post-partum depression and seasonal affective disorder (SAD)

Depression can occur during pregnancy, with a peak of incidence between weeks 18 to 32 of gestation, but most cases of depression happen soon after delivery of the baby. **Post-partum syndrome** occurs in some women at any time from 3 days to 6 weeks after giving birth. The cause is unknown, but a hormonal imbalance, stress or a genetic predisposition to mood disorders have all been suggested as contributing factors. About one-third of all sufferers have a previous history of a psychiatric disorder and about one-quarter will have more than one episode. Some women may show signs *before* the birth which suggest that a depressive illness could follow labour; such signs include lack of preparation for the baby, denying the pregnancy or expressing future plans that clearly do not involve the baby. The range of severity is wide, from a mild form (often called *baby blues*) to an intense suicidal psychotic depression.

- *Post-partum blues*, a mild depression that lasts 1 to 14 days after the birth, often peaking on the fifth day, in which the new mother feels low and cries easily. She may show hostility towards the baby or even the father.
- *Post-partum depression*, a more severe syndrome occurring at any time up to 6 months after the birth and which lasts for most of the first year. These mothers show loss of emotion, anxiety, reduced appetite, sleep

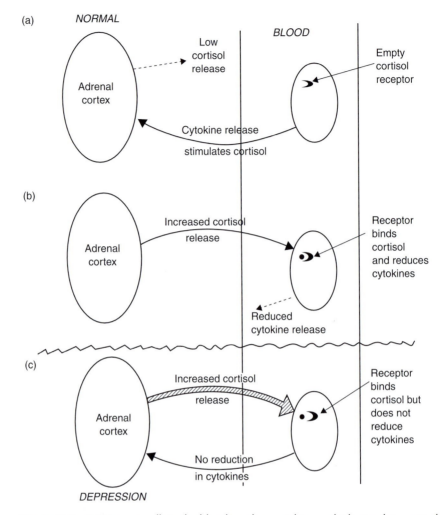

FIGURE 9.6 (a) Immune cells in the blood produce cytokines, which stimulate cortisol production when this is low. (b) As cortisol levels rise, cortisol binds to cortisol receptors in the immune cells and this reduces cytokine production. (c) In depression, the receptors do not function so well, resulting in continued cytokine production when cortisol level is high.

disturbance and guilty feelings. Most of the women have no intentions of harming themselves or the baby.

- *Post-partum psychosis*, the most severe form, in which the mother loses contact with reality and show signs of psychosis (hallucinations, delusions and disorientation). The depression takes the form of unipolar or bipolar depression, with harmful tendencies towards the baby (who may be seen as the cause of their problem) or themselves.

Seasonal affective disorder (SAD) is a depressive state that occurs during the winter months when shorter days are accompanied by less sun, i.e.

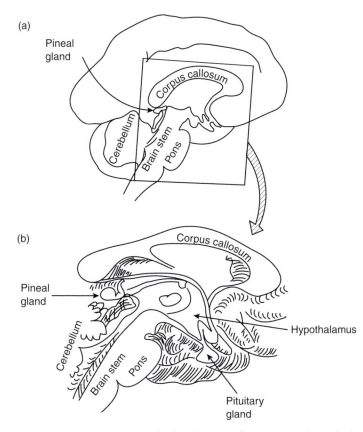

FIGURE 9.7 Location of the pineal gland. (a) Midline section through the brain, view from the right. (b) Close-up of the upper brain stem, hypothalamus and corpus callosum, showing the pineal gland.

when light levels are lower. Serotonin is used by the **pineal gland** (found immediately behind the hypothalamus, Figure 9.7) to make a hormone called **melatonin**. **Pinealocytes** (cells of the pineal gland) concentrate serotonin, which is then converted first to **N-acetylserotonin**, then to melatonin. Melatonin can cross membranes better than serotonin and it binds to receptors to form complexes that interact with cellular activity. The pineal gland is sensitive to light levels on the retina (part of the retinal output to the brain goes to the pineal gland via the hypothalamus, the **retinohypothalamic tract**). During the dark, noradrenaline levels rise and this acts on the pineal gland to create melatonin from serotonin. Melatonin may be the true trigger of sleep, as it is involved in the normal sleep–wake cycle, which is clearly driven by the external cue of changing light levels. Melatonin levels are very low during the day when noradrenaline levels are lower. The winter months of long nights and lower daytime light levels can maintain a higher than expected melatonin level and this may trigger a persistent depressive mood throughout winter. SAD can sometimes be treated with artificial light (called **phototherapy**) (Birtwistle and Martin 1999).

The antidepressant drugs

The main neurotransmitters involved in depression are the *monoamines* serotonin and noradrenaline (Blows 2000a,b). The **monoamine hypothesis** of depression came from two important observations made in the 1950s:

- Some patients treated for hypertension with a drug called **reserpine** were becoming depressed.
- Some patients treated for tuberculosis with a drug called **para-amino salicylic acid (PAS)**, were becoming happier.

Reserpine was later found to deplete the synapses of both their serotonin and noradrenaline, thus inducing a depressive state. PAS, however, was noted to block the enzyme that breaks down the neurotransmitter, thus allowing the neurotransmitter to increase in the synapse and therefore relieving depression. The enzyme concerned is **monoamine oxidase**, which is found in association with the mitochondria of the presynaptic bulb. After use in the synaptic cleft, many neurotransmitters are returned to the presynaptic bulb *See page 32* (*re-uptake*) for conversion to a **metabolite** before removal from the brain. This creates two possible mechanisms for increasing the amounts of neurotransmitter in the synaptic cleft:

- Blocking the re-uptake so that the chemical stays in the cleft. This is the principal mode of action of the **tricyclic antidepressants** and *some* **atypical antidepressants**.
- Blocking of the breakdown by inhibiting the enzyme so that the chemical stays in the synapse. This is the principal mode of action of the **monoamine oxidase inhibitors (MAOI)**.

Tricyclic antidepressants

These drugs are named after the three-ringed (*tri-cyclic*) nature of the their chemistry, known as the **dibenzazepine** structure (Figure 9.8a). They work by blocking the re-uptake of the neurotransmitters serotonin and noradrenaline into the presynaptic bulb, with the result that these transmitters accumulate in the synaptic cleft. Two of the drugs in early use were **amitriptyline** (Figure 9.8a), which has approximately equal activity in blocking both neurotransmitters, and **imipramine**, which is more selective in blocking noradrenaline. Other typical tricyclic antidepressant drugs are **doxepin**, **nortriptyline**, **protriptyline** and **trimipramine**.

This drug group had the problem that symptoms of depression were not relieved until up to two weeks into treatment. This was difficult to understand; after all, the very first dose of the drug given was active in raising the neurotransmitter levels at the synapse, so why was mood taking so long to return to normal? Worse still, during this two-week delay, the patient was acquiring more energy and a severely depressed patient with more energy was a greater suicide risk. There had to be another mechanism by which these drugs were relieving depression and another way round this

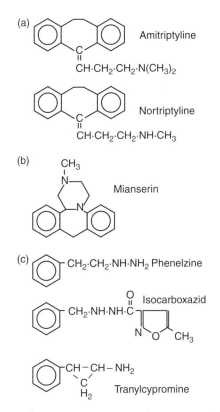

FIGURE 9.8 Structure of some important antidepressants: (a) tricyclic drugs; (b) atypical drugs; (c) monoamine oxidase inhibitor (MAOI) drugs.

delay. One step forward was the development of drugs which were more selective for blocking the re-uptake of either serotonin (the **serotonin-selective re-uptake inhibitors**, or **SSRI**) or noradrenaline (Table 9.4).

The side-effects of the tricyclic antidepressants are drowsiness, dry mouth, blurred vision, urinary retention and constipation, all of which are **antimuscarinic** effects. Muscarinic receptors bind the neurotransmitter acetylcholine. Muscarine is a plant alkaloid that binds to this receptor, thus giving its name to the receptor. As antagonists, the tricyclic antide-pressants prevent acetylcholine from binding to muscarinic receptors, and in this way cause the side-effects. Other side-effects include **hypona-traemia** (low blood sodium levels) in the elderly and occasionally **cardiac arrhythmias** (abnormal rhythms of heart activity) such as **heart block** (failure of electrical conduction through the heart). The most likely tricyclic drug interactions are with the MAOI drug group. The switching of treat-ment from tricyclic to MAOI, or from MAOI to tricyclic medication, should only be done after a time gap of two weeks or more. The SSRI drugs have fewer antimuscarinic side-effects and appear to be less problematic to the heart. They do, however, sometimes cause varying degrees of nausea and vomiting.

See page 59

See page 196

TABLE 9.4 Selective serotonin and noradrenaline inhibitors

Serotonin-selective re-uptake inhibitors	Noradrenaline-selective inhibitors
Fluoxetine	Maprotiline
Citalopram	Viloxazine
Sertraline	Nomifensine
Paroxetine	Nortryptiline
Fluvoxamine	Reboxetine

TABLE 9.5 Some atypical antidepressants

Atypical antidepressant	Notes
Mirtazapine	Blocks presynaptic α_2-adrenoceptors, which causes an increase in noradrenaline release
Mianserin (Figure 9.8b)	Reduces sensitivity of postsynaptic β-adrenoceptors (which alters the balance of postsynaptic adrenoceptor activity); it also blocks presynaptic α_2-adrenoceptors, which causes an increase in noradrenaline release
Nefazodone	Serotonin re-uptake inhibitor but selectively blocks some serotonin receptors, thus altering the balance of which receptors serotonin binds to

Atypical antidepressants

These drugs are newer derivatives of the tricyclic group (Figure 9.8b). While some do block the re-uptake of neurotransmitter at the synapse, others do not. The fact that they relieve depression without interfering with the re-uptake of neurotransmitter adds weight to the notion that blocking re-uptake is not the primary mechanism for relieving depression. These drugs, either exclusively or partially, modify the function of serotonin or noradrenaline receptor sites (Table 9.5) and this gives a clue as to the mechanism by which all antidepressant drugs ultimately work. Drugs of this atypical group appear to relieve symptoms faster than the tricyclic drugs and they are known to be active in the limbic areas of the brain. Because many of them do not block transmitter re-uptake, they tend to cause fewer side-effects than the tricyclic group.

Monoamine oxidase inhibitors (MAOI)

The introduction of MAOI drugs (Figure 9.8c) that block the enzyme monoamine oxidase was one of the earliest treatments available for depression. Monoamine oxidase is an enzyme located on the outer membrane of mitochondria in the presynaptic bulb, particularly in the dopaminergic, adrenergic and serotonergic pathways. The enzyme inactivates the neurotransmitter after it has done its work in the synaptic cleft and has been taken back into the bulb. When the enzyme is blocked with the inhibitor drug, the neurotransmitter cannot be reduced to its metabolites for excretion and remains in the synapse. The transmitter levels then rise in the bulb and cleft. This action is more pronounced in noradrenergic and serotonergic synapses than in doperminergic synapses.

Two forms of MAO exist, MAO-A and MAO-B, but the human brain has mostly MAO-B. Both forms of the enzyme degrade all three neurotransmitters (dopamine, noradrenaline and serotonin) when these transmitters are in high concentration, but when they are in lower concentrations the enzymes become more specific. Both forms of the enzyme also exist in many tissues outside the brain, in particular the gut wall and the liver. The purpose of having the enzyme in these digestion-related sites is to facilitate the degradation of monoamines found in the diet, mostly **tyromine**. If tyromine enters the blood unmodified by MAO it can cause a hypertensive crisis. A throbbing headache is an early sign of this potentially dangerous condition. This is what happened to some patients given MAOI drugs for depression before it was realised that dietary monoamines were the cause of their crisis. To allow continuation of the treatment with the MAOI drugs it became necessary to remove monoamines from the diet. Patients were then issued with a list of foods to avoid, particularly those that contain the monoamine tyromine: foods such as cheese, pickled herring, red wine, and yeast or meat extracts to name a few. On the surface, it does seem paradoxical to issue potentially suicidal patients with tablets and a list of foods that may, in combination, kill them! In reality, of course, it was more selective and controlled than this picture would suggest, with potentially suicidal patients admitted for observation. However, occasional fatalities did occur and it became apparent that this was not the ideal way to cope with the problem.

All the original MAOI drugs worked by the *irreversible* blocking of the enzyme MAO, which meant that the enzyme had to be degraded, removed and replaced by a new enzyme. The problem of potentially dangerous hypertensive crisis led to the development of the newer *reversible* MAOI (RIMA) drugs. These work by locking on to and inhibiting the enzyme when the monoamine levels are low, thus allowing the levels to accumulate and rise. Should there be a sudden rise in monoamines – for example, in the digestive tract following the eating of a cheese sandwich – the drug will unlock from the enzyme, which then becomes free to act on the monoamines in the diet. Meanwhile, the same drug will remain active in the brain where the monoamine levels are low, thus exerting its antidepressant qualities. The action of the drug is therefore dependent on the amine levels in the area where it is found. As a result, the presence of monoamines in the diet has become a less important issue, although patients should still avoid consuming large amounts of these foods. The only such RIMA drug currently available in clinical practice is listed in Table 9.6, but others may follow. No two antidepressants should be prescribed for the same patient at the same time and, as with the tricyclic antidepressants, MAOI must not be started immediately after tricyclic drugs. At least two weeks should be allowed before commencing the MAOI after stopping the tricyclic drug. This is

TABLE 9.6 MAOI antidepressants (Figure 9.8c)

Irreversible MAOI drugs	Reversible MAOI drugs (RIMA)
Phenelzine	Moclobemide (MAO-A specific)
Isocarboxazid	Caroxazone (MAO-B specific)[a]
Tranylcypromine	

[a] The drug is in development and not yet in clinical practice.

because of the potentially hazardous interactions that can occur between these drug groups.

MAOI drugs can cause side-effects such as **postural hypotension** (low blood pressure on standing up from a sitting or lying position, a particular problem for elderly patients on these drugs) and dizziness. Other noted side-effects include dry mouth, drowsiness, insomnia, headache, fatigue, gastrointestinal disturbances, difficulty with **micturition** (passing urine) and many more, some potentially serious. For all these reasons, MAOI drugs are usually a second-line choice of treatment, used when the tricyclic or atypical drugs have failed.

If, as has been seen, the relief of depression is not (at least not entirely) dependent on the increase in neurotransmitter levels in the brain, how do antidepressants really work? The full answer remains unknown. The current thinking is that all the antidepressant drugs work to relieve depression by two possible mechanisms:

- re-adjustment of the sensitivity of the receptors for serotonin and noradrenaline;
- modification of the transport of these neurotransmitters across the presynaptic membrane.

It seems likely that depression is the result of defective neurotransmitter transporter and receptor activity at the synapse, and that the abnormal levels of neurotransmitter are a consequence of this. The antidepressants work to correct these defects and in so doing readjust the HPA axis to normal at the same time. Tricyclic and MAOI drugs take about 14 days to achieve this, but some of the atypical drugs can begin to relieve the symptoms earlier.

Mood-stabilising drugs

The drugs described under this heading are those used to prevent the swings in mood associated with bipolar depression, in which long periods of deep depression are interrupted by occasional bouts of mania. **Lithium carbonate** is very effective in this role by controlling the manic state when used in a prophylactic manner. It has no role to play in the management of unipolar depression.

See page 181

Lithium is given orally and is rapidly absorbed from the gut, peak levels being reached in the blood within 24 hours of commencement. The mechanism by which lithium balances mood is not entirely understood, partly because several biochemical effects occur together, and deciding which results in the desired effect is difficult to determine. Lithium is a **cation** (a positively charged particle) and can act as a substitute for other cations such as sodium (Na^+), potassium (K^+), magnesium (Mg^{2+}) or calcium (Ca^{2+}). Lithium can penetrate the neuronal cell body membrane and accumulate within the cytoplasm. This increases the intracellular cation population, repelling some K^+, which is forced out of the cell. This results in a partial *depolarisation* of that neuron, and in turn slows the *repolarisation* phase, thus reducing the excitation of the neuron. Lithium has several other effects:

- It inhibits **ATPase** (the enzyme that produces **ATP, adenosine triphosphate**, the cell's high-energy molecule), causing a reduction in the level of ATP in the cell.
- It has a similar inhibitory effect on **cAMP (cyclic adenosine monophosphate)** and **inositol**. *See page 42*
- It slows down the uptake of choline into the neurons that synthesise acetylcholine and this neurotransmitter is therefore reduced.
- It causes reduced release of serotonin and reduced serotonin receptor density in the hippocampus.
- It prevents dopamine receptors in the corpus striatum from becoming supersensitive to dopamine, a possibility that can occur after long-term use of the **neuroleptic** drugs. This particular action of lithium is probably quite an important mechanism leading to the desired antimanic effect. However, there are several other effects in the brain that make it difficult to pinpoint the exact antimanic action of lithium.
- It has significant antiviral effects, especially against the **herpes virus**.
- It has modulatory effects on cell-mediated and humoral immunity. This suggests a possible role for viral infections in depression. *See page 189*

Toxic levels of lithium are achieved rapidly if the dose is not carefully controlled and blood levels are not monitored. The effects, which may be worsened by a low blood sodium level, include tremor, **ataxia** (unsteady walking), nausea, dizziness, convulsions and coma. Lithium can also cause a wide range of other side-effects, such as endocrine disturbance, notably **thyroid disorders**, by inhibiting iodine uptake into the thyroid gland and reducing thyroid hormone production. Alterations of the thyroid receptor concentration in the hypothalamus as a result of lithium treatment may have some bearing on its mood-stabilising role given the importance of the thyroid for brain activity. It also can cause **polyurea** (a large urine output) with **polydipsia** (excessive thirst), weight gain, oedema and gastrointestinal disturbances. Changes in the electrical rhythm of the heart may be noticed on the **electrocardiogram** (**ECG**). Clearly, the decision to use lithium is not taken lightly, and usually involves specialist advice. *See page 65*

Carbamazepine is also available for the prophylaxis of mania, especially in those patients who are unresponsive to lithium. It is particularly useful in patients who have a rapid cycle of manic and depressive episodes (i.e. four or more such episodes per year). This drug is an important anti-epileptic and as such is discussed in Chapter 10.

Key points

Depressive illness

- Depressive illness occurs when the depressed state has no apparent cause or when the period of depression is prolonged beyond what is considered normal.
- Two main types of illnesses occur, unipolar depression (depression only) and bipolar depression (symptoms of depression with periods of mania).

Risk

- For the population as a whole, the risk of developing unipolar depression is 6%, and for bipolar depression the risk is 1%.
- First-degree relatives of a bipolar depressed patient have a concordance rate of 19%, while for unipolar depression the concordance rate is 10%.
- The concordance rate for bipolar depression in monozygotic twins is about 65%; in dizygotic twins the concordance rate is about 14%. This indicates that bipolar depression is a genetically based disease.

Cause

- Genes on chromosomes 11, 18, 21 and X have all been implicated.
- An X-linked form of bipolar disorder has been located to Xq28 (major affective disorder 2, or *MAFD2* gene).
- Environmental factors appear to play a much bigger role in the aetiology of unipolar than of bipolar depression.

Brain pathology

- Between 10% and 30% of depressed patients have some ventricular enlargement, and some patients show a reduction in the size of the temporal lobe.
- Reduced blood flow to the left anterior cingulate gyrus and the left dorsolateral prefrontal cortex has been identified.
- Symptoms of mood disorder are most likely to arise with dysfunction of the temporal and frontal lobecortex plus either the temporal lobe-associated limbic areas or the pathway from the basal ganglia to the cortex via the thalamus.

Biochemistry and immunity

- Serotonin is reduced and a low turnover of the transmitter occurs at the synapse. Very low levels of serotonin have been linked to increased violent behaviour, such as suicide. Serotonin is used by the pineal gland to make the hormone melatonin.

- The serotonin subtype-2 receptor (5-HT2) is thought to be the most important receptor involved in mood regulation.
- A low serotonin level causes a lower noradrenaline level in the brain.
- There is a disturbance in the numbers and density of noradrenaline receptors in depression.
- Severe bipolar depression with psychotic symptoms may be due to disturbance of the dopaminergic systems.
- A prolonged hyperactivity of the hypathalomo–pituitary–adrenal (HPA) axis occurs, causing chronic CRF (corticotropin-releasing factor) and cortisol release. There are also indications of dysfunction of the hypathalomo–pituitary–thyroid (HPT) axis, causing thyroid hormones abnormalities.
- There are significant immune system changes in depression.

Post-partum depression

- Post-partum depression, in which women become depressed after birth, is an umbrella term for three conditions: post-partum blues (a mild depression), post-partum depression (a more severe syndrome) and post-partum psychosis (the most severe form).

SAD

- Seasonal affective disorder (SAD) is a depressive state occurring during the winter months when there are shorter days and low light levels.

Tricyclic antidepressants

- Tricyclic antidepressants work by blocking the re-uptake of serotonin and noradrenaline into the presynaptic bulb, so these transmitters accumulate in the synaptic cleft.
- Some tricyclics are more selective for either serotonin (serotonin-selective re-uptake inhibitors, or SSRI) or noradrenaline.
- The side-effects of tricyclic antidepressants are caused by their antimuscarinic activity.

Atypical antidepressants

- Atypical antidepressants modify the function of serotonin or noradrenaline receptor sites.

MAOI antidepressants

- Monoamine oxidase inhibitors (MAOI) block the enzyme monoamine oxidase, which normally breaks down neurotransmitters.

- Antidepressant drugs relieve depression mainly by re-adjusting the sensitivity of the receptors for serotonin and noradrenaline, and by modifying the transport of these neurotransmitters across the presynaptic membrane.
- MAOI drugs require restriction of oral intake of the monoamine tyromine to prevent hypertensive crisis.
- Different antidepressant drugs should not be prescribed without at least a two-week gap between them to prevent drug interactions.

Lithium

- Lithium is a prophylactic mood-stabilising drug used to control the manic phases of bipolar depression. Lithium can reach toxic levels quickly and must be carefully monitored.

References

Birtwistle J. and Martin N. (1999) Seasonal affective disorder: its recognition and treatment. *British Journal of Nursing*, **8** (15): 1004–1009.

Blows W. T. (2000a) Neurotransmitters of the brain: serotonin, noradrenaline (norepinephrine), and dopamine. *Journal of Neuroscience Nursing*, **32** (4): 234–238.

Blows W. T. (2000b) The neurobiology of antidepressants. *Journal of Neuroscience Nursing*, **32** (3): 177–180.

Brown P. (1997) No way out. *New Scientist*, 22 March: 34–37.

Brown P. (2001) A mind under siege. *New Scientist*, **170** (2295; 16 June): 34–37.

Carlson N. R. (2001) *Physiology of Behavior* (7th edn). Allyn and Bacon, Boston.

Mestel R. (1997) Mind altering bugs. *New Scientist*, 13 Sept.: 42–45.

Nemeroff C. B. (1998) The neurobiology of depression. *Scientific American*, June: 28–35.

Ron M. A. (1999) Psychiatric manifestations of demonstrable brain disease, *in* Ron M. A. and David A. S. (eds), *Disorders of Brain and Mind*. Cambridge University Press, Cambridge.

Thompson C. (1996) Mood disorders. *Medicine*, **24** (2): 1–6.

Wild G. C. and Benzel E. C. (1994) *Essentials of Neurochemistry*. Jones and Bartlett, London.

Chapter 10

Epilepsy

Seizures: types and causes

Epilepsy is a term used to cover a very wide range of complex disorders, all characterised by the presence of seizures or fits and sometimes convulsions. **Seizures**, or **fits**, are brief periods of altered consciousness accompanied by changes in sensory and motor function, causing momentarily abnormal behavioural patterns. The altered state of consciousness may mean a short period of either total or partial loss of consciousness, or simply a state of unawareness. **Convulsions** are powerful, often violent, rhythmic muscular contractions of the trunk and limbs occurring during a seizure. The word **ictal** is used to indicate a fit, with **interictal** meaning the period between two successive fits. Seizures occur in a variety of major or minor types.

Generalised seizures

Generalised seizures are characterised by unconsciousness due to spread of an electrical discharge to many areas of the brain and they are often associated with convulsions. They account for about 30% of all epilepsies. *Generalised epilepsies* can be classified into four types: **absences**, **generalised tonic–clonic**, **myoclonic** and **atonic**. Of these four types, the first two are the most common.

Absence (formally the **petit mal** or **minor fit**) describes a transient loss of awareness during which the person will stop what they are doing, stare vacantly into space for about 30 seconds or so, perhaps fumble with objects around them, then return to normal. There is no perceptive or cognitive function for the duration of the fit and afterwards there is no memory of the event. The person does not fall to the ground because normal **muscle tone** is maintained. Occasionally **automatism** (mechanical automatic movements) is seen, particularly if the duration of the fit is longer than 30 seconds. Petit mal usually starts at around the age of 5–7 years and stops at puberty. **Atypical absences** show a similar clinical picture, but the person may also show muscle twitching or some other abnormal movement. This form of seizure usually lasts longer than the typical absence and is probably more common (Russell and Hanscombe 1997).

Generalised tonic–clonic fits (the **grand mal** or **major fit**), are those in which the person loses consciousness, falls to the ground and convulses. This form of epilepsy is the type most people think of as a fit in the true sense of the word. Such fits occur in three ways: as *primary generalised epilepsy*, where there is no other neurological abnormality; as a *partial seizure* which becomes generalised; and as a symptom associated with *diffuse brain dysfunction*.

Myoclonic fits (**myo** = muscle, **clonus** = rapid, alternating contractions and relaxations of skeletal muscle) are those in which muscle jerks occur in the arms or legs for a short period of about 1–5 seconds. Atonic (a = without, tonic = tone, also called **drop attacks**) fits are those in which there is a sudden loss of muscle tone, resulting in collapse of the person. They last only a few seconds.

Partial (or focal) seizures

Focal seizures are centred around one particular part of the brain with some spread of the impulses, but spread is more limited than in generalised seizures. This is the most common type of seizure. In the abnormal physiology of partial seizures the neurons fire rapid bursts of action potentials which are then synchronised in other neuron groups as the wave of impulses spreads.

Consciousness is often preserved (**simple partial**), but sometimes lost (**complex partial**) depending on the cause of the seizure, the location of the initial site and the spread of the electrical impulse. Behavioural changes are often a feature. The areas of the brain usually involved are:

TABLE 10.1 The known causes of seizures

Cause of seizures	Notes
Congenital defects	Caused by disruption to neuronal function
Head injury (accidental or birth)	From brain damage or raised intercranial pressure (RICP)
Brain tumours and CNS disorders	Caused by disruption to neuronal function
Intercranial infections	Caused by irritation of the brain surface
Febrile	Caused by high temperature in children under 7 years of age
Drugs and alcohol withdrawal	Caused by removal of depressive effect on neuronal function
Metabolic	Caused by disturbance of neuronal biochemistry
Psychological	Invented by the patient for a specific purpose

- *Frontal lobe*. Seizures originating here cause predominantly motor symptoms, especially of the legs and the head. These seizures last for just a few seconds and occur several times a day.
- *Parietal lobe*. Seizures originating here can cause sensory and motor symptoms as in **Jacksonian epilepsy**. See page 216
- *Temporal lobe*. Seizures originating here cause personality symptoms, as typified in **temporal lobe epilepsy**. See page 215
- *Occipital lobe*. Seizures originating here cause disturbance of the visual cortex, resulting in the patient seeing visual phenomena such as flashing lights or sparks.

Fits are either of known or unknown aetiology. The designation unknown probably means that the underlying pathology remains undetected. Those caused by known pathology are listed in Table 10.1.

Idiopathic, or **primary epilepsy** (indicated as **1°**) is of unknown cause; that is, the existing pathology cannot be explained, and may be due to a developmental malformation of the brain structure. **Symptomatic**, or **secondary epilepsy** (indicated as **2°**) is caused by distinct and explainable brain pathology, either in structure or function. There are also various syndromes involving fits (Table 10.2) and special forms of epilepsy (see text for temporal lobe and Jacksonian epilepsy).

The electroencephalogram (EEG) in epilepsy

The EEG is a very useful tool in the investigation of epileptic syndromes but it cannot be used alone to diagnose epilepsy. It does have a value in helping to distinguish between the different categories of epilepsy. Basically, the EEG is a recording of the overall pattern of electrical signals generated by millions of active neurons across the brain surface. A characteristic epileptic feature on the EEG is the *spike*, a pointed feature in the wave pattern not seen on the normal tracing, as shown in Figure 10.1. During seizures the

TABLE 10.2 Special syndromes and forms of epilepsy

Special epileptic syndromes	Notes
West syndrome (generalised)	Involves infant developmental delay, muscle spasms and long-term intellectual handicap
Lennox-Gastaut syndrome (generalised)	Multiple tonic or atonic seizures per day, sometimes absences, drop-attacks or myoclonus. Slow mental development or even intellectual regression with learning difficulties. Caused by nerurodevelopmental abnormalities or brain injury
Kojewnikow's syndrome (partial)	Partial motor seizures followed by myoclonic jerks. Some neurological deficits
Landau–Kleffner syndrome (generalised)	Acquired aphasia (speech loss). Two-thirds have seizures and/or behavioural and intellectual problems
Myoclonic epilepsy and ragged red fibres (MERRF)	Seizures with myopathy (muscle deterioration) (see text)

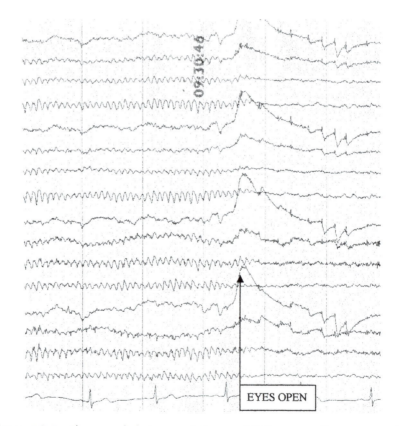

FIGURE 10.1 The normal electroencephalogram (EEG) tracing. There is no 'spike' feature often seen in epilepsy.

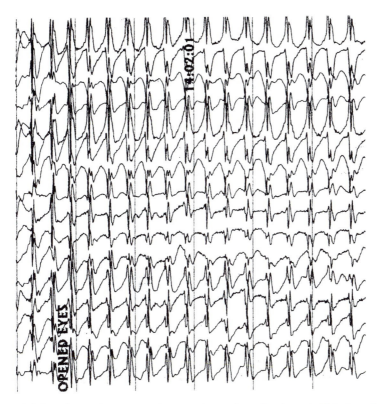

FIGURE 10.2 The EEG seen in absences (or petit mal seizures). This is a 3-per-second wave pattern.

wave patterns and spikes show increased frequencies and abnormal irregularities as the seizure spreads. The following patterns are usually seen.

- Absences show a 3-per-second spike and wave activity (Figure 10.2).
- Simple partial seizures show localised slow but sharp wave activity (Figure 10.3).
- Complex partial seizures show a medium-voltage spike activity centred on one brain area, increasing in intensity as it spreads (Figure 10.4).
- Generalised tonic–clonic seizures show rhythmic high-voltage activity leading to the clinical appearance of convulsions, with bilateral multispiked wave patterns during convulsions (Figure 10.5).

Factors involved in the cause of epilepsy

It is estimated that the total number of people in the United Kingdom who have ever had a fit is about 5% (including febrile convulsions). The occurrence of one fit does not mean the sufferer has epilepsy and of this 5% group only about 0.5% will go on to develop true epilepsy after their first fit. Fits are basically the result of **cerebral irritation**, meaning anything that directly disturbs the function of neurons in the brain, and the majority

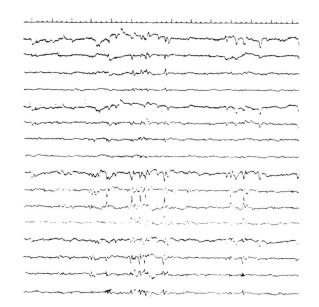

FIGURE 10.3 The EEG seen in simple partial seizures.

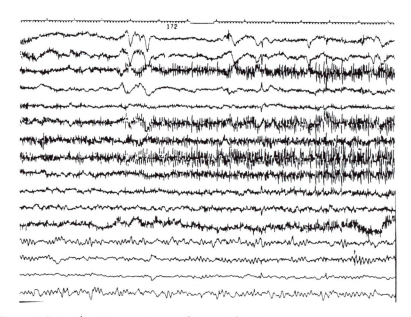

FIGURE 10.4 The EEG seen in complex partial seizures.

of these *one-off* fits are caused by temporary self-correcting or curable problems.

Age. The incidence of fits increases with age; 12 per 100 000 people between 40 and 59 years of age are affected and this figure rises to 80 per 100 000 in the population over 60 years. One-quarter of the epileptic population is over 60 years old.

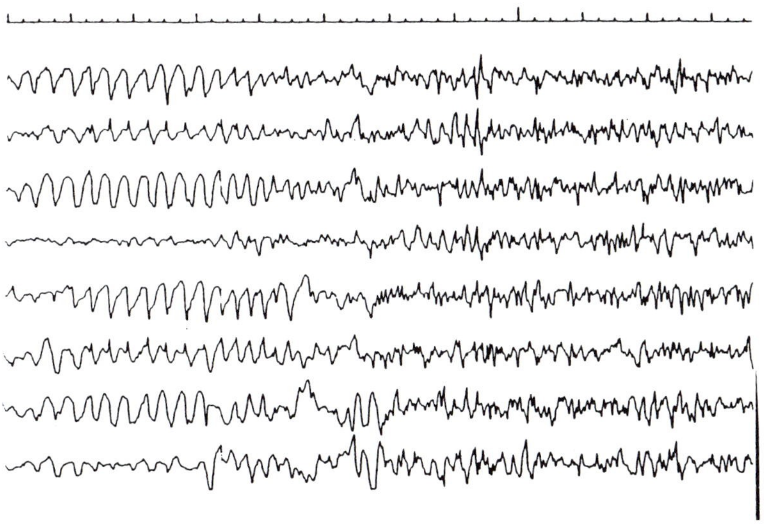

FIGURE 10.5 The EEG seen in general tonic–clonic (or grand mal) seizures.

Genetics. Epilepsy can be familial, but the picture is often complicated by the effects of several genes involved acting together (polygenic), or by varying amounts of genetic penetrance. There are close to 150 rare genetic disorders that have an increased risk of epilepsy as a common feature. Of these, about 100 are **autosomal recessive**, 25 are **autosomal dominant**, and the remainder are **X-linked**. Examples include autosomal genes found at chromosome loci 6q (**juvenile myoclonic epilepsy**), 8q (**progressive epilepsy with mental retardation**), 20q (**benign familial neonatal convulsions, or BFNC**) and 21q (**progressive myoclonus epilepsy, or PME, or Unverricht–Lundborg disease**) (see Table 10.3) (Treiman and Treiman 1996). Others are likely to be discovered with the advances expected in human genetics over the next decade or so.

See page 76

Not all the genes responsible for epilepsy are found in the karyotype. DNA, the molecular basis of genes, is also found in **mitochondria**, the cellular organelles charged with the task of energy production. Mitochondria need their own genes to code for the proteins involved in the energy cycle. One mitochondrial gene mutation that can cause seizures is **MERRF (myoclonic epilepsy and ragged red fibres)** (Figure 10.6). The 'ragged red fibres' are the accumulations of mitochondria seen on biopsy below the cell membrane of skeletal muscle. A change from the DNA base adenine to guanine in the normal gene causes a mutation that reduces mRNA production and thus protein synthesis. Skeletal muscle then deteriorates and the person becomes deaf and demented before the seizures and myoclonus and ataxia begin (Wallace 1997).

Tonic–clonic (grand mal) seizures

A number of epileptic fits are caused by an **epileptogenic focus** (Hickey 1997; McCance and Huether 1994). This is a lesion at a specific site in the

TABLE 10.3 Autosomal-linked epilepsies

Autosomal-linked epilepsy	Notes
Juvenile myoclonic epilepsy	Myoclonus while awake, absence seizures, plus generalised tonic–clonic seizures in early teens
Progressive epilepsy with mental retardation	Generalised tonic–clonic seizures begin at 5 to 10 years of age, increasing until puberty, and then declining in frequency to 35 years, when the person remains seizure-free. Mental deterioration begins about 5 years after seizures begin and requires nursing care
Benign familial neonatal convulsions (BFNC)	Seizures from 2nd or 3rd day after birth cease at about 6 months of age. Development after that is normal
Progressive myoclonus epilepsy (PME) (Unverricht–Lundborg disease)	Appears between 6 and 15 years of age; tonic–clonic seizures, gradual intellectual decline leading to ataxia, tremor and dysarthria

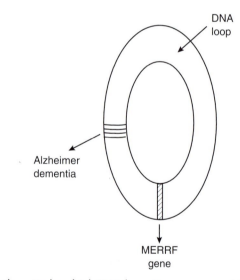

FIGURE 10.6 The mitochondrial DNA loop. Two genes on this loop are important for mental health, one associated with Alzheimer's dementia, and the myoclonic epilepsy and ragged red fibres (MERRF) gene, which causes a syndrome that includes epilepsy.

brain where, as a result of damage or changes in their biochemistry, the neurons periodically give off abnormal discharges that spread to other parts of the brain and cause a fit. It is useful to think of a fit as an electric *storm* in the brain spreading from one particular point. Where the epileptogenic

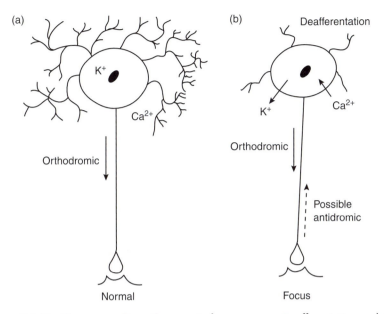

(a)   (b) Deafferentation

K+

Ca²⁺

Orthodromic

Orthodromic

Normal

K+   Ca²⁺

Possible antidromic

Focus

Figure 10.7 Changes at the epileptogenic focus neuron. Deafferentation, calcium entry, and possible antidromic impulses are some of the features that cause greater electrical activity at the focus.

focus is known and has been studied, several interesting characteristics have been found (Figure 10.7):

- The neurons of the focus may suffer some degree of **deafferentation**, i.e. a loss of dendrites, the afferent component of the neuron. The reason for this is not fully understood, but it causes a chronic state of depolarisation and excitability in the neurons (Groer and Shekleton 1989). *See page 24*
- The normal passage of an action potential is from the cell to the synapse, and this is described as an **orthodromic** impulse. There is some evidence to suggest that the epileptogenic focus can sometimes generate **antidromic** impulses, which return abnormally from the synapse back up the axon. This is probably one reason for a rapid depolarisation in the axon of the focal neurons. The antidromic impulses may also generate other orthodromic impulses, creating a cycle. This cycle of impulses up and down the first (focal) axon could cause repeated orthodromic impulses to pass out to the body and may be part of the mechanism for creating the rhythmic convulsions.
- The focal neurons have reduced GABA activity; i.e. less inhibition from the GABA neurons. They also show disturbed protein metabolism. *See page 48*
- Calcium (Ca²⁺) is normally in greater concentrations outside the neuronal cell body, with potassium (K⁺) inside. During a seizure, focal neurons leak calcium *into* the cell and this displaces potassium *out of* the cell. These ionic changes cause further hyperexcitability of the neuron (Groer and Shekleton 1989).

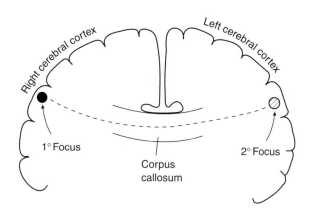

Figure 10.8 The primary focus (1°) sometimes causes a secondary focus (2°) to form at the mirror image position on the other side of the brain. They link through the corpus callosum. Removal of the primary focus causes the secondary focus to disappear.

- Occasionally, an epileptogenic focus is present in one hemisphere of the brain (either cortical or subcortical), but a second focus can be traced in the mirror image site in the other hemisphere (Figure 10.8) (Hickey 1997; McCance and Huether 1994). The true focus is **primary** (**1°**) and communicates with the false **secondary** (**2°**) focus through the corpus callosum. The secondary focus is essentially normal brain tissue acting along with the true focus to cause the seizure. Removal of the primary focus, as is possible in some patients, results in the normalisation of the secondary focus.

The net effect of all these changes at the epileptogenic focus is to produce a small area of neurons which are hyperactive with a low threshold for firing impulses. They are likely to discharge action potentials easily and rapidly, up to 1000 impulses per second during a fit, sparking off a wave of abnormal electrical activity across the brain. Each impulse is seen as a spike on the EEG. Lateral spread to the cerebral cortex and the brain stem is responsible for the loss of consciousness, and downward spread to the body may cause the convulsive events.

During a fit the brain increases its use of ATP (adenosine triphosphate) as an energy source by 250%. This huge energy requirement must be met by an increase in the blood supply, which also increases by 250%. The oxygen consumption of the neurons increases by 60%, but still this massive supply becomes depleted. The brain moves into anaerobic metabolism, with the result that lactic acid production, acidosis and cellular exhaustion occur (McCance and Huether 1994). Fits rarely last for more than a few minutes. It is thought that the fit stops either because the neurotransmitters are depleted or because the rapid accumulation of waste products, including lactic acid, cannot be removed fast enough. In either case any further neuronal activity would be prevented.

Generalised tonic–clonic fits are not due to an epileptogenic focus but are caused by a more widespread irritation of brain cells. Some factors that lead

TABLE 10.4 Stages of a grand mal fit

Stage of the fit	Notes
1. **Aura**, or warning	Occurs in the form of confusion, aggression, or hallucinations such as flashing lights or strange smells. Many patients do not have an aura
2. **Tonic**	Fall to the ground followed by increased muscle tone which causes arching of the body on the ground. Lasts about 15–30 seconds, during which breathing stops and the patient becomes somewhat cyanosed
3. **Clonic**	The convulsive stage. The patient thrashes about. They may be incontinent. Breathing is spasmodic and excessive salivation causes frothing at the mouth. Lasts for about 30–60 seconds
4. **Recovery**	Starts when the patient stops moving. Breathing gradually settles down. Patient goes from unconsciousness into sleep, and then wakens. They may be a little confused or disorientated. There is no memory of the event. Lasts about 5–10 minutes or so

to this form of grand mal seizure are listed in Table 10.1. This is why those having an epileptic-type fit for the first time must undergo extensive investigations to identify the presence or absence of a focus and, if the latter, what may be the cause.

Table 10.4 describes the main stages and features of this form of epilepsy. Table 10.5 indicates the nurse's role at each stage of the fit.

Some myths related to what to do during a fit are explored here.

• The placing of a hard object between the teeth to stop the person from biting their tongue is usually done *too late* and therefore becomes a dangerous procedure. By the start of the tonic phase the jaw will be clenched tightly shut, and to open the jaw would require a considerable force, causing injury to the patient's mouth. Bleeding into the mouth and dental damage would cause a further risk of airway obstruction and distress when the patient wakes up. If the person is going to bite their tongue, this will have happened by the start of the tonic phase. This means that the aura is the only stage at which it is possible to take preventive action. Since an aura does not always occur, and if it does it is over very quickly, it is probably best to relegate this procedure to the history books.

• The restraining of the body during the convulsion is another very dangerous practice. Anyone attempting this is putting themselves and the patient at considerable risk of injury, and it is unnecessary. The patient's limb movements are powerful, and they may kick, punch or throw off anyone holding them. In addition, it has been shown that restraint causes more limb injuries to the patient than allowing them to be free. Emptying

TABLE 10.5 Nurse's skill at each stage of the fit

Stage of the fit	Nurse's (or first-aider's) role at each stage
1. **Aura**	Assist the patient to the ground in a clear area to avoid injury when falling or convulsing. Loosen tight clothing neck, chest and waist. Note the time
2. **Tonic**	Work from the head end away from the body. Do not restrain the patient. Keep other people away from the patient's body. Keep the airway as clear as possible. Do not try to put anything between the teeth as this will cause oral damage and bleeding into the mouth. Clear the area around the patient
3. **Clonic**	Continue to work from the head end away from the body. Do not restrain the patient. Observe and facilitate breathing by clearing the airway of any obstruction. Check the pulse (carotid is best) and skin colour for cyanosis
4. **Recovery**	Turn into the recovery position when convulsion stops. Stay at head end to maintain clear airway and check breathing, pulse and skin colour. On the patient's awakening, get them into a resting position gradually. Note the time again

the space around the patient's body to give them room is a useful thing to do, to prevent them hitting against hard objects. Everyone should keep clear of the patient's body, while the nurse stays at the head end.

The **recovery stage** is an important time for nursing care. The patient should be placed in the *recovery position* as soon as the clonic phase ends. The nurse should remain with the patient at all times, unless there is no choice but to leave to get help. If going to get help is the only choice, leave the patient in the *recovery position*. The patient may go into a second fit, so the nurse should remain to assist should this happen. Staying at the head end, the nurse should *maintain a clear airway* and *observe for breathing, pulse and cyanosis* (blue colour of the skin, indicating a lack of oxygen). Check the patient's *level of consciousness* every few minutes by talking to them (Blows 2001). On return to consciousness, allow the patient time to rest, reassure them, and help them orientate themselves to time, place and what happened. The patient can sit up *slowly*, when ready to do so. The nurse should make a note of the time at each stage of the fit, but especially the time taken for recovery. A prolonged time of the recovery phase, i.e. longer than 30 minutes, may be a sign of complications. Be aware of the possibilities of complications and seek help if required. Some of the possible complications are:

- The patient may go into another fit. If this happens then they must receive urgent medical care to prevent further fitting. **Status epilepticus** is a very serious complication in which patients continue to fit for up to 24 hours or more. It is dangerous because patients can die from exhaustion or heart failure and prolonged convulsions create a shortage of oxygen to the brain, causing brain damage.

- **Postepileptic (interictal) twilight state** is a prolonged period of confusion and disorientation following a fit. Restless wandering and abnormal behaviour can accompany a twilight state. Patients do not know what they are doing and may unknowingly carry out bizarre, dangerous and even criminal acts. Again, urgent medical help is needed to safeguard the patient.

Temporal lobe seizures (psychomotor epilepsy)

Epilepsy caused by temporal lobe lesions has a specific set of characteristics. The main occurrence is an abrupt change in personality and restless automatic behaviour patterns, with or without a concluding loss of consciousness. Hallucinations of an **olfactory** (smell) or **gustatory** (taste) nature sometimes occur and the patient may experience **déjà vu**, i.e. the sense of events repeating themselves, or **jamais vu**, the sense of being a stranger in familiar company or environments. Psychotic symptoms can present, with aggressive overtones, and emotional or mood swings. This sudden change in the behaviour and personality can be very frightening to the witness, who is often a member of the patient's family, and the nurse's support is needed to allay their fears. The sudden onset of the symptoms and the quick return to normal are strong indications that the cause is a seizure, even in the absence of convulsions.

The temporal lobe lesion responsible is often **medial temporal sclerosis**, a hardening of the temporal brain tissue, which occurs often in the hippocampus, notably that part called **Ammon's horn** (see the anatomy of the hippocampus). This lesion is associated with cerebral anoxia, especially as a fetus, or can result from febrile convulsions early in childhood, particularly if they were complicated or prolonged. The child grows up free from seizures for many years, but then develops temporal lobe epilepsy in early adulthood.

See page 165

One part of the temporal lobe is the *limbic portion* (i.e. the area that connects and works with the limbic system), and epilepsy caused by a lesion here is referred to as **medial temporal epilepsy syndrome** (or simply **limbic epilepsy**). Again, the characteristics of this syndrome involve behavioural difficulties and psychotic, schizophrenia-like symptoms. There is also an **interictal syndrome** (i.e. symptoms occurring between fits), identified by reduced sexual behaviour, increased religious convictions (e.g. compulsive church attendance) and **hypergraphia** (excessive compulsive writing). The presence of psychosis as part of an epileptic illness is confusing, since without the fits these patients may well be diagnosed as schizophrenic. Often this raises the question: *Does the epilepsy cause this psychosis*, or, *Is this a schizophrenic illness with the patient having fits as well?* One suggested distinction between the 'psychosis of epilepsy' and the 'psychosis of schizophrenia' is that the former is a milder psychosis with fewer negative symptoms, no thought disorder, preservation of affect and a distinct increase in religious delusions (Trimble 1999).

Jacksonian seizures

Jacksonian fits begin with a unilateral twitching of muscles in one part of the body – for example, the small finger of the *left* hand and from there the convulsion spreads to all other parts of the same side of the body, and then onto the other side. The patient becomes unconscious and has a full convulsion. The muscles involved at the start indicate which part of the cerebral motor cortex was generating the fit, i.e. the focus of the lesion. In our example, the lesion would be in the *right* motor cortex (Brodmann 4), the area that controls the little finger. Notice that the *right* motor cortex controls the *left* side because most of the motor fibres cross in the brain stem. The lesion in the motor cortex could be a tumour, inflammation or scar tissue. Keen observation by the nurse can pinpoint the muscles involved at the start of the twitching and thereby assist the doctor in the diagnosis.

Infantile spasms and febrile convulsions

Infantile spasms (or **hypsarrhythmia**) are attacks of head nodding and flexing of the body that begin in the early months of life. Gross abnormalities of the brain are one cause of this form of epilepsy and in this case it can lead to progressive mental retardation. However, another cause is a deficiency of **vitamin B$_6$ (pyridoxine)** in the diet and treatment simply involves replacing the vitamin.

Infantile (or febrile) convulsions are not true epilepsy and very few cases go on to develop epilepsy later in life. The cause is a high temperature in children below the age of 7 years when the temperature control centre in the hypothalamus is still immature. Prevention of the convulsion can sometimes be achieved by the administration of **paracetamol** in syrup form when the child is conscious and able to swallow, during the early stages of a raised temperature. Nursing measures include reducing clothing, cooling the *room* (not the child directly) with a fan, or tepid sponging. If consciousness is lost and convulsions commence, do not attempt to give any further oral medication. Maintain a clear airway, continue cooling the child and seek medical assistance as quickly as possible (Blows 2001).

The anticonvulsant drugs

The several classes of drugs used in the treatment of epilepsy act in two main ways: on the epileptogenic focus to prevent discharge from happening; or on the brain as a whole to prevent spread of the discharge. There are a number of different means of achieving these functions (Figure 10.9):

- *Sodium channel blockers* act by blocking the channels through which sodium influxes the axon during an action potential. This prevents the action potential from travelling any further down the axon and the discharge is blocked from spreading. In this way these drugs stabilise the axonal membrane. The drugs in this group are **phenytoin, carbamazepine** and **sodium valproate.**

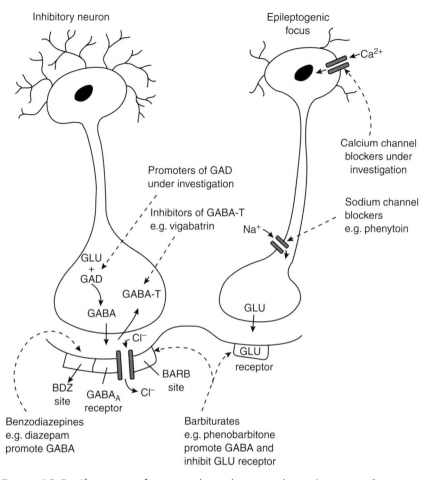

FIGURE 10.9 The action of anticonvulsant drugs. At the epileptogenic focus (top right) calcium enters abnormally and excites the cell. Calcium channel blockers may be useful to prevent cell excitation. The abnormal action potentials (impulses) from the focus pass down the axon where sodium influxes. Blocking the sodium channels would halt the progress of the impulses. At the synapse, glutamate is released. Blocking the glutamate receptor will halt the impulses at that point. The inhibitory neuron (top left) produces gamma-aminobutyric acid (GABA), which blocks impulses. Promoting glutamic acid decarboxylase (GAD) or inhibiting GABA-transaminase (GABA-T) will increase the level of GABA at the synapse. Drugs that increase GABA activity at the $GABA_A$ receptor will help to inhibit abnormal impulses.

- Other drugs *promote GABA activity* by binding to the $GABA_A$ receptor complex (Figures 3.13 and 10.9). This enhances the action of GABA, which opens the chloride channels and causes inhibition of any further action potentials, preventing spread of the discharges across the brain. The drugs in this group are the **benzodiazepines** (e.g. **diazepam**, **clonazepam** and **lorazepam**, which are used in several types of epilepsy) (Table 10.6) and the **barbiturates** (**phenobarbitone** is the drug of this group used in epilepsy). Increasing the amount of GABA available

See page 48

See page 110

TABLE 10.6 Drugs used in specific epileptic categories

Epileptic category	Drugs used in the treatment
Partial seizures	
Simple	Carbamazepine, sodium valproate, phenytoin
Complex	Carbamazepine, sodium valproate, phenytoin
Generalised seizures	
Absences	Ethosuximide, sodium valproate, clonazepam
Tonic–clonic	Carbamazepine, sodium valproate, phenytoin, or phenobarnitone
Myoclonic	Sodium valproate, clonazepam, ethosuximide
Status epilepticus	Diazepam, clonazepam, lorazepam, paraldehyde, phenytoin (preventive)
Infantile spasms	Clonazepam, also effectively treated with ACTH
Infantile (febrile) convulsions	Diazepam

in the brain is another way of improving inhibition of action potentials; the drug **sodium valproate** achieves this by preventing the GABA breakdown metabolism after use, so that the neurotransmitter builds up in quantity at the synapse.

See page 48

- Phenobarbitone also *suppresses glutamate activity*, glutamate being the excitatory neurotransmitter of the cerebrum. Suppressing the excitatory action of glutamate will reduce the ability of the abnormal discharge to spread across the cerebrum. This drug is especially useful in having a dual role in combating the spread of seizures.

See page 211

- *Calcium channel blockers* have been tried as anticonvulsant therapy, with some success in clinical trials. They prevent the influx of calcium into the neuron cell body and this reduces the ability of the epileptogenic focus to discharge action potentials. The drugs in this group are currently undergoing trials and may be released for clinical use in the future.

Particular drugs are used to treat specific epileptic syndromes, as indicated in Table 10.6.

Side-effects of the anticonvulsant drugs are quite extensive and relate to the specific drugs listed in Table 10.6. Sedation is a problem with some drugs, notably the benzodiazepines and phenobarbitone, and this may cause difficulties with some activities. Phenytoin side-effects are numerous, including dizziness, nausea, skin rashes, insomnia and gastrointestinal disturbance, **nystagmus** (rapid, involuntary flicking of the eyes), **ataxia** (unsteady walking) and **diplopia** (double vision). However, it still has a valuable contribution to make to anticonvulsive therapy. Carbamazepine and ethosuximide both have similar lists of extensive side-effects, including headache, dizziness, drowsiness, ataxia and gastrointestinal problems. More serious side-effects, such as **agranulocytosis** (reduced white blood cell counts), **aplastic**

anaemia (low red blood cell counts due to reduced bone marrow activity) and even mental depression are less often reported. Sodium valproate can cause nausea, ataxia, gastric irritation, tremor, increased appetite and weight gain, transient hair loss and occasional blood disorders. This drug can also be toxic to the liver and can disturb the blood clotting mechanism, so careful patient selection and persistent monitoring of blood clotting and liver function are important.

Drug interactions are also a problem and this is a good reason for patients to be given **monotherapy**, i.e. treatment with one drug only. The patient is unlikely to benefit from several drugs at once and toxic effects can occur quickly, with an unpredictable outcome. Care must be taken to ensure that the anticonvulsant drug prescribed is compatible with any other form of medication the patient may be taking. Check with the drug interaction information in the prescription handbooks. Withdrawal of any anticonvulsant drug must be done slowly, with staged reductions in dosage. This particularly applies to the benzodiazepines and barbiturates. Abrupt withdrawal of the drug, or sudden change of one drug to another, may cause *rebound seizures* to occur.

Key points

Types of seizures

- Generalised fits are characterised by unconsciousness; partial (or focal) seizures, are centred around one particular part of the brain with limited spread.
- Generalised fits include absences, and generalised tonic–clonic, myotonic and atonic seizures.
- Partial fits may be simple (no loss of consciousness) or complex (loss of consciousness).
- Idiopathic, or primary, epilepsy is of unknown cause and may be due to a developmental malformation of the brain structure. Symptomatic, or secondary, epilepsy is caused by distinct and explainable brain pathology.
- Types of fits include absence (formally the petit mal, or minor fit), where there is a transient loss of consciousness (10–15 seconds) and generalised tonic–clonic (the grand mal, or major fit), where the patient loses consciousness, falls to the ground and convulses.

Electroencephalogram

- EEGs have value in helping to distinguish between the different categories of epilepsy.

Factors involved in the cause of epilepsy

- The incidence of fits increases with age.
- Epilepsy can be familial; about 100 epileptic disorders are autosomal recessive, 25 are autosomal dominant, and the remainder are X-linked.

- Many epileptic fits are caused by an epileptogenic focus, a lesion at a specific site in the brain that can trigger a fit.
- The neurons of the focus appear to suffer some degree of deafferentation, abnormal glucose and protein metabolism, reduced GABA activity and the production of an orthodromic–antidromic loop during a seizure.
- Focal neurons also have abnormal calcium influx, and calcium channel blockers may be another future form of therapy.
- The primary focus is sometimes linked to a secondary focus in the opposite hemisphere, which disappears if the primary is removed.

Tonic–clonic (grand mal) seizures

- The four phases of a grand mal fit are aura (if present), tonic, clonic and recovery.
- Nurses should not force anything between the patient's teeth during a fit.
- Nurses should never restrain a convulsing patient.
- Work from the head end during a fit to clear the airway and maintain observations.
- Place the patient in the recovery position when the recovery stage begins.
- Get help if complications arise, such as in status epilepticus or postepileptic twilight state.

Temporal lobe seizures

- Temporal lobe epilepsy (or psychomotor epilepsy) is characterised by an abrupt change in personality and restless automatic behaviour patterns, with or without a concluding loss of consciousness.
- The lesion is medial temporal sclerosis, a hardening of the temporal lobe brain tissue, often in the hippocampus.
- Medial temporal epilepsy syndrome (limbic epilepsy) involves pathology of the limbic-associated areas of the temporal lobe.
- Interictal syndrome (symptoms occurring between fits), involves reduced sexual behaviour, increased religious convictions and hypergraphia.

Jacksonian seizures

- Jacksonian fits begin with a unilateral twitching of muscles in one part of the body, and it spreads from there to all other parts of the body.

Anticonvulsant drugs

- Benzodiazepine and barbiturates act by binding to the $GABA_A$ receptor and promote the opening of the GABA-mediated chloride channels to inhibit any action potentials.
- Phenytoin, sodium valproate and carbamazepine are sodium channel blockers, blocking the entry of sodium into the axon during an action potential.

- Monotherapy is preferred to prevent drug interactions and toxicity.
- Withdrawal of anticonvulsants should be gradual.

References

Blows W. T. (2001) *The Biological Basis of Nursing: Clinical Observations*. Routledge, London.

Groer M. W. and Shekleton M. E. (1989) *Basic Pathophysiology, A Holistic Approach*. Mosby, St Louis.

Hickey J. V. (1997) *The Clinical Practice of Neurological and Neurosurgical Nursing* (4th edn). Lippincott, Philadelphia.

McCance K. L. and Huether S. E. (1994) *Pathophysiology, The Biological Basis for Disease in Adults and Children* (2nd edn). Mosby, St Louis.

Russell A. and Hanscomb A. (1997) Epilepsy: the most common serious neurological condition. *Nursing Times* **93** (21): 52–55.

Treiman L. J. and Treiman D. M. (1996) Genetic aspects of epilepsy, *in* Wyllie E. (ed.), *The Treatment of Epilepsy: Principles and Practice*. Williams and Wilkins, Baltimore.

Trimble M. R. (1999) A neurobiological perspective of the behaviour disorder of epilepsy, *in* Ron M. A. and David A. S. (eds) *Disorders of Brain and Mind*. Cambridge University Press, Cambridge.

Wallace D. C. (1997) Mitochondrial DNA in aging and disease. *Scientific American* Aug.: 22–29.

Chapter 11

Subcortical degenerative diseases of the brain

- Introduction: the basal ganglia
- Parkinson disease
- The anti-Parkinson drugs
- Huntington disease
- Wilson's disease and Harvey's disease
- Key points

Introduction: the basal ganglia

The subcortical degenerative diseases, often called the **subcortical dementias**, are included here because, like the cortical dementias (Chapter 12) they sometimes fall into the care of the psychiatric nurse. The reason is that they are often associated with depression and psychoses (Kaplan and Sadock 1996). These disorders are essentially caused by degeneration of the basal ganglia, those parts of the brain below the conscious cortex that have a powerful influence over body movements and muscle tone (Aird 2000). The basal ganglia form part of a loop that regulates motor function. This loop starts with the **frontal cortex**, which projects fibres to the **corpus striatum**. The striatum has connections with both the **globus pallidus** and the **substantia nigra pars reticulum**, which then connect to various nuclei of the **thalamus**. Finally, the thalamus connects back to the frontal lobe, completing the loop (Figure 11.1). Degeneration of any part of this loop can cause both motor symptoms (basal ganglia) and psychotic symptoms (frontal lobe). Central to the production of symptoms in these disorders is the disturbance to

See page 11

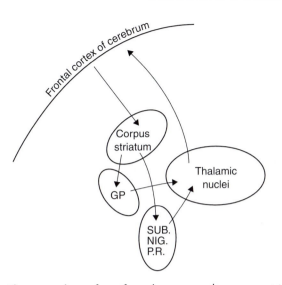

Figure 11.1 The motor loop, from frontal cortex to the corpus striatum, then to both the globus pallidus and the substantia nigra pars reticular (SUB. NIG. P.R). From here the connection is with the thalamus then back to the cortex.

dopamine metabolism. Dopamine depletion in the basal ganglia causes motor deficits, while dopamine depletion in the frontal lobes generates cognitive and psychotic symptoms.

The basal ganglia are five separate nuclei of neuronal cell bodies (see Figure 1.7). The main pathways between the nuclei and their connections with other brain areas are as follows (Figure 11.2). The **caudate nucleus** and the **putamen** (together called the **corpus striatum**) have an input from the cerebral cortex (the *higher centres* of the brain) that involves the neurotransmitter **glutamate**. Two outputs from the caudate nucleus to the **globus pallidus** use GABA as the neurotransmitter; one is an excitatory pathway to the **medial globus pallidus (GP$_m$)**, the other is an inhibitory pathway to the **lateral globus pallidus (GP$_l$)**. The putamen has an output to part of the **substantia nigra** called the **pars reticulata** (abbreviated to **SN$_r$**). The other part of the substantia nigra, the **pars compacta (SN$_c$)**, has dopaminergic feedback loops to both components of the corpus striatum, i.e. an excitatory loop back to the putamen, an excitatory loop back to the GP$_m$ caudate nucleus output, and an inhibitory loop back to the GP$_l$ caudate nucleus output. The output from GP$_l$ to the **subthalamic nucleus (STN)** utilises GABA, while the outputs from the STN to both the SN$_r$ and the GP$_m$ are facilitated via glutamate. Both the SN$_r$ and the GP$_m$ have GABA-mediated outputs to the **thalamus** (Bear *et al.* 1996). All these pathways can be visualised using Figure 11.2. From Chapter 1 we recognise that *the substantia nigra is responsible for lowering muscle tone and it does this through its dopaminergic pathways to the corpus striatum.* This statement is fundamental to our understanding of Parkinson's disease.

See page 12

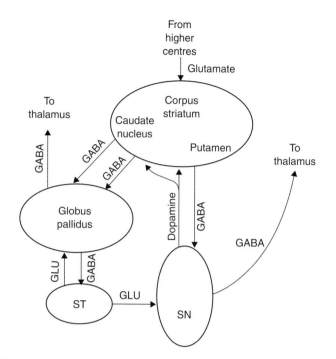

FIGURE 11.2 Normal basal ganglia pathways. Compare with Figure 11.3. GLU = glutamate; GABA = gamma-aminobutyric acid; SN = substantia nigra, ST = subthalamus.

Parkinson disease (PD)

James Parkinson (1755–1824) was a general practitioner working in Shoreditch, East London, not far from the Royal London Hospital at Whitechapel in East London. He noticed a number of people with a strange stiffness to their gait and shaking limbs. The term used to describe this was **paralysis agitans** (*agitated paralysis* or *shaking palsy*) and it only became known as Parkinson's disease (PD) at a later date. PD affects about 2 people per 1000 in the UK population.

Muscle stiffness (or **rigidity**) and shaking of the limbs (or **tremor**) have become the classic signs of the disease. The major features of Parkinson's disease are therefore as follows.

- Progressive muscle rigidity due to increasing muscle tone. The body and limbs become stiff and movement is very limited (i.e. an **akinesia** = a muscular paralysis, or a **bradykinesia** or **hypokinesis** = slow voluntary movements) (Borrell 2000) causing difficulty in initiating movement, which is sometimes known as **freezing**. These are often relieved during sleep.
- Shaking of the limbs, both *coarse* tremors of the whole limb and *fine* tremors of the hand and fingers. These are reduced during intentional movement of the limb, but become very marked at rest. Fine tremors of

the hand are sometimes called *pill rolling*, because they resemble the hand movements used to roll pills before the days of quality control.

- People with PD adopt a forward stance, i.e. leaning slightly forwards, and walk with a shuffling gait. When walking, the top half of the body tends to move forwards faster than the feet, and there is a risk of falling forwards onto the face. In one study, 59% of people with PD had falls, and of these falls 49% resulted in injuries (Gray and Hildebrand 2000). Factors that increase the risk of falling were identified as the severity of the symptoms of the disease, the effectiveness of the medication, the activities and the location of the person at the time of the fall and the degree of fatigue they were suffering at the time (Gray and Hildebrand 2000).

- The arms are held in a bent fashion, in a position similar to that seen in the insect called a praying mantis.

- The facial muscles are paralysed by the excessive muscle tone and this results in the inability to adopt a facial expression, known as the **Parkinsonian mask**.

- Speech becomes difficult and is reduced to a low, mumbled and hurried voice that is almost impossible to understand.

- The mouth tends to hang open and produce excessive saliva (called **sialorrhoea**). This results in patients dribbling saliva down their front. Having one's mouth open all the time is embarrassing, so patients often try to solve both these problems by putting a handkerchief in their mouth. The handkerchief soaks up the excess saliva and blocks the open mouth.

- Swallowing becomes difficult as the disease progresses and towards the latter stages nasogastric tube feeding may be required.

- The patient's handwriting becomes impossible to read and communication with the patient becomes very difficult.

- **Oculogyric crisis** is a phenomenon that occurs perhaps several times a day. The eyes rotate upwards so that the iris is hidden under the upper lid and they are held there for a minute or so before returning to normal. This muscular spasm of the eye muscles is said to be very painful.

- Other associated symptoms include constipation, sexual dysfunction, **orthostatic** or **postural hypotension** (low blood pressure on standing), and bladder dysfunction due to disturbance of the **autonomic nervous system** (i.e. the component of the nervous system that maintains automatic organ functions) (Herndon *et al.* 2000). Observations by the nurse during their day-to-day management of the patient may identify specific autonomic problems which will need to be addressed.

- Sleep disturbances occur often in PD and the nurse is in the best position to be able to assist the patient and to advise the family concerning interventions that promote adequate rest (Crabb 2001).

- Psychiatric symptoms can occur, such as **depression** (up to 16.5% of PD patients) and **hallucinations** (up to 37% of PD patients) and these require specific management (Herndon *et al.* 2000). Nurses need to be alert to this and report any symptoms of depression (e.g. sleep disturbance) or **psychosis** that they observe.

225

- **Dementia** has been identified in as many as 25% of patients with PD (Herndon *et al.* 2000), further complicating both the clinical appearance of the disease and its management.

What is happening in this disorder is that, for reasons that remain unknown, the substantia nigra is gradually degenerating, neurons of this nucleus are dying and are not being replaced. Since the function of the substantia nigra is to lower muscle tone (and the function of the cerebellum is to increase muscle tone), there is normally a balance between the two. The gradual loss of the substantia nigra upsets that balance in favour of the cerebellum (which remains normal). Muscle tone therefore increases unopposed, but the symptoms only become apparent quite late in the disorder because the deterioration of the substantia nigra is very slow and because the neurons are able to compensate to some extent for the losses. Symptoms do not usually appear until the substantia nigra has lost 60% of its cells (Roberts *et al.* 1993), so that patients diagnosed with Parkinson's disease have had the disorder for many years without symptoms. This is one reason why the disease usually affects those over 60 years of age, although occasionally it is seen in some patients earlier in life. The substantia nigra (which means 'black substance') is so called because its neurons contain a large quantity of **neuromelanin**, a pigment that gives the cells a dark coloration. As these cells die in Parkinson's disease, the neuromelanin is released, and antibodies in the blood that are specific to neuromelanin are increased. This increase *may* prove to be useful as a test in the early detection of the disease long before symptoms arise (Nowak 2000).

See page 254

In addition to cells losses, affected cells also develop **Lewy bodies**. These are intracellular collections of neurofilamentous material (i.e. made of neurofilaments) surrounding a central core of proteins, fatty acids and polysaccharides. The cause of these bodies and their effect on the cells are still not clear, although it seems that affected cells are likely to degenerate and die. In Parkinson's disease, the substantia nigra is the main site of Lewy body formation, although they can sometimes be identified in other parts of the brain, for example in the cortex when dementia or psychoses also occur. Lewy bodies are also seen in a variety of other neurological disorders, notably in dementia.

See page 247

As part of their role, the neurons of the substantia nigra pars compacta (SN_c) produce dopamine, but the loss of cells in Parkinson's disease means that the SN_c becomes unable to produce dopamine. Within the pathway that extends from the substantia nigra to the corpus striatum, i.e. the **nigrostriatal pathway**, dopamine levels drop very low. The symptoms of the disease are related to this effect (Figure 11.3), but there is a threshold of 80% loss of dopamine in this pathway before symptoms occur. Clearly a loss of 80% dopamine takes a very long time to achieve.

See page 44

The gradual loss of the doperminergic nigrostriatal pathway has a knock-on effect on the remaining basal ganglia (follow these steps by comparing Figure 11.2 with Figure 11.3):

- Low dopamine excitation from the SN_c to the putamen results in lower GABA activity from the putamen to the SN_r. This reduced

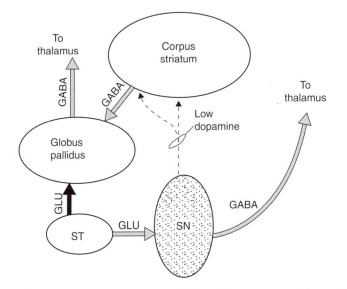

FIGURE 11.3 In Parkinson's disease, the lack of dopaminergic pathways from the dying substantia nigra (shown dark) to the corpus striatum causes increased GABA activity in the other pathways shown. The result is excess motor disturbance to the thalamus. (Abbreviations as in Figure 11.2.)

GABA inhibition of SN_r allows an increased GABA inhibition of the thalamus.

- Low dopamine inhibition from the SN_c to the caudate nucleus allows an increase in the GABA inhibitory effect from the caudate nucleus on GP_l. GP_l inhibition is increased, causing lower GABA inhibition of the subthalamus (STN).

- The loss of the inhibitory effects of GABA from the GP_l on the STN allows the STN to increase the excitatory glutamate pathways to both the GP_m and the SN_r, and thus cause increased GABA inhibition of the thalamus.

- Low dopamine excitation from the SN_c of the caudate nucleus reduces the caudate nucleus GABA activity to GP_m. This results in a low caudate nucleus GABA inhibition of the GP_m. The GP_m is now free to increase its own GABA inhibition of the thalamus.

- The thalamus is now receiving increased GABA inhibition from both the GP_m and the SN_r, causing inhibition of the thalamus is its vital motor role.

The cause of the disease is unknown although two factors are emerging as candidates:

- *Genetics.* Genes for Parkinson's disease are now being traced, indicating that some people have a genetic predisposition for developing the problem. These people include certain family groups and those presenting with symptoms at less than 50 years of age. Mutations of the alpha-**synuclein**

227

See page 226

gene are found in some PD families and the alpha-synuclein protein is also found in Lewy bodies. Other gene mutations have been traced to 2p13 and 6q25.2–27, but the genetic involvement of the majority of sporadic cases of PD remains unclear.

- *Environment.* A neurotoxin has been identified that induces the disease in animals, but also in those humans who have accidentally made contact with it. The neurotoxin is called **N-methyl-4-phenyl-1,2,3, 6-tetrahydropyridine**, (or **MPTP**). Some drug addicts in America injected this substance into themselves by mistake and developed advanced, irreversible Parkinson's disease. MPTP probably works by being changed first to **1-methyl-4-phenylpyridinium** (**MPP⁺**) by the action of the

See page 197

enzyme MAO-B. By interfering with the energy cycle within the mitochondrion, and by inducing the formation of damaging chemical agents called **superoxide radicals**, MPP⁺ is more neurotoxic than its precursor MPTP. As such, the presence of MPP⁺ results in depleted energy levels, neural damage and cellular losses (Figure 11.4). The discovery of MPTP has opened the way to new research that may lead to a better understanding of this disease. Questions still need to be answered, such as *How do ordinary people who have never taken illegal drugs, or their related chemicals, get exposure to MPTP?* Some possible neurotoxins acting against the basal ganglia are suspected, mostly in form of pesticides used in the agricultural industry. An alternative observation may also account for the energy losses in these neurons. Deletions of some mitochondrial DNA, i.e. the genes that code for enzymes of the energy chain within the mitochondria, have been found in some Parkinson's disease patients. Loss of these genes would result in the failure of energy production within the neuron, leading to cell death (Figure 11.4). Mitochondrial DNA mutations are known to be a factor in the cause of

See page 247

Alzheimer disease (a form of dementia), and **Leigh syndrome** (a progressive loss of movement and speech due to basal ganglia degeneration in children).

The anti-Parkinson drugs

It might sound reasonable to treat Parkinson's disease by simply replacing the missing neurotransmitter with dopamine, thus restoring the muscle tone balance between the substantia nigra and the cerebellum. There are two main problems with this scenario:

- Dopamine does not cross the blood–brain barrier and, moreover, dopamine outside the brain (in general circulation) causes unpleasant side-effects.
- Simply replacing dopamine does not stop the relentless deterioration of the substantia nigra, the main cause of the symptoms, so this can never be a cure.

Nevertheless, this notion of replacing dopamine in order to improve the quality of life has become the mainstay of treatment. Since dopamine could

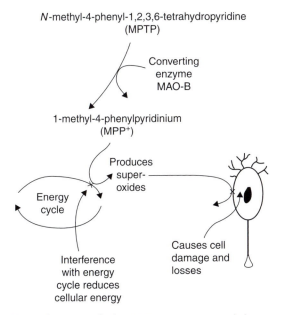

FIGURE 11.4 The pathway in which MPTP causes neuronal damage and losses.

not be given directly, the precursor called **levodopa** (L-**dopa**), which does cross the blood–brain barrier, was used. Conversion from levodopa to dopamine is made in the neurons of the basal ganglia. Remember, however, that the dopaminergic neurons of the substantia nigra are slowly dying, so their ability to convert levodopa to dopamine is in gradual decline. In the 1960s, the use of levodopa was shown to have dramatic effects in relieving symptoms. Some decades on, it has become clear that levodopa has some serious long-term problems:

- The amount of conversion of levodopa to dopamine in the brain is completely unpredictable. While the dose of levodopa administered can be controlled, what happens after that is less controlled. The same levodopa dose can have different results on different days. A way around this problem is to give the minimum dose in combination with other drugs. *See page 231*
- The amount of conversion of levodopa to dopamine declines with time. After 5 years of treatment with levodopa, the patient needs higher dosages to achieve a reasonable result. Higher dosages mean more side-effects. One cause of this is that dopamine receptors are losing their sensitivity and more neurotransmitter is needed to stimulate them. A way around this is to give the patient a **drug holiday**. This means removing them from all their medication (except antibiotics if they happen to be on them) for about 2–4 days. During this drug-free time the patient suffers the full symptoms, but the dopamine receptors are re-sensitised and on reinstatement of levodopa the patient will become symptom-free on a lower levodopa dosage.

- The enzyme that converts levodopa to dopamine, called **dopa decarboxy-lase**, is found also in other tissues outside the brain, so part of the levodopa dose is converted to dopamine in the body. Of course, once converted to dopamine it cannot cross the blood–brain barrier. So the dopamine levels in circulation build up, causing side-effects. To prevent this, another drug, called a **dopa-decarboxylase inhibitor**, is given to block the enzyme *outside* the brain (but *not inside* the brain since the inhibitor cannot cross the blood–brain barrier) so that the levodopa enters the brain and is converted there. These inhibitor drugs are **benserazide** and **carbidopa**. In modern Parkinson's disease therapy, the inhibitor drug is given built into the levodopa; for example, benserazide with levodopa is called **co-beneldopa**, and carbidopa with levodopa is called **co-careldopa**.
- Some patients suffer the **on–off phenomenon**, which means the sudden switching from a near symptom-free state to severe symptoms, and back again, several times throughout the day. This gets worse as the length of the treatment period increases. The sudden nature and severity of this switching is distressing, but can be reduced by splitting the dose from once per day to several times throughout the day. This gives a better regulation of blood levels of levodopa, and improves the control of symptoms.
- **End of dose deterioration** means that the period of symptom-free benefit after each dose becomes progressively shorter. A change to *modified-release* preparations, from which levodopa is released slowly over a longer time span, can help to overcome this problem.

The side-effects of levodopa are anorexia, nausea, dizziness, **tachycardia** (fast pulse rate), **arrhythmias** (abnormal changes in heart rhythm), insomnia and **postural hypotension** (low blood pressure when standing upright).

Other drugs

See page 60
See page 16

Antimuscarinic drugs – drugs that are antagonistic to (or block) the acetyl-choline muscarinic receptors – work by preventing the activity of the para-sympathetic nervous system and therefore allow the sympathetic nervous system to become dominant. This group of drugs includes **benzhexol**, **orphenadrine** and **procyclidine**. They are less effective than levodopa, but are useful in reducing some symptoms, notably the sialorrhoea (excess of saliva). They also facilitate some decrease in rigidity and tremor.

Dopamine agonists are drugs that act like dopamine in the brain and stimulate dopamine receptors. However, since they are not dopamine they have no problems crossing the blood–brain barrier and require no enzyme conversion. The drugs in this group include **bromocriptine**, **carbergoline**, **lisuride** and **pergolide**. They can be used to augment the role of levodopa in patients in whom either levodopa alone is inadequate or it becomes diffi-cult to control blood levels. They can help to prevent the *on–off phenomenon*. Some side-effects, such as nausea, vomiting, headaches, dizziness, hypoten-sion, drowsiness and confusion limit their use. **Ropinirole** is a D_2 receptor agonist and **pramipexole** is an agonist for both the D_2 and D_3 receptors. **Apomorphine** is a D_1 and D_2 receptor agonist which is useful in the management of the *on–off phenomenon*.

Modern treatment of Parkinson's disease is tailor-made to suit the patient, because so many factors are involved, such as the patient's age, stage of the disease and drug reactions. Many patients are treated with a combination therapy of some levodopa together with the enzyme-inhibiting drug, and perhaps another additional drug given as an adjunct therapy to overcome the problems of levodopa.

Huntington disease (HD)

George Huntington (1850–1916) was an American doctor in general practice. He was the son and grandson of doctors and all three of these men had noticed the strange symptoms, known as **chorea**, that this disease produced in several American families. In 1872, at the age of just 21 years, George Huntington published a paper in which these patients were briefly described. The affected families, ultimately involving about 1000 patients occurring over 12 generations, were centred on the east end of Long Island, New York. They could trace their ancestry back to two brothers in Sussex, England, indicating the strong genetic basis of this disorder. The origins of the gene mutation are not clear, but it may have first occurred centuries ago in East Anglia, England, and is now widely disseminated across the world.

Huntington disease (HD) is a neurodegenerative disorder of the basal ganglia, notably the caudate nucleus first, followed by the putamen (i.e. the corpus striatum), with concurrent enlargement of the lateral ventricles (Figure 11.5) (Carlson 2001). The disorder starts to produce symptoms between the ages of 30 and 45 years, in other words usually after the affected

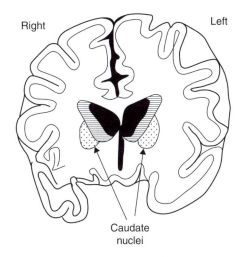

Right — Left

Caudate
nuclei

FIGURE 11.5 Huntington disease. Section through the brain showing the size of the normal ventricles (in black) and the increased size of the ventricles (shown by the cross hatched area) in Huntington disease due to destruction of the caudate nuclei.

person has had their family and has passed the affected gene to the offspring. Up to 10 years prior to the onset of movement disorder, a number of patients show mild psychotic and behavioural symptoms, possibly due to the stress of living in a family with a genetic problem. A reduced cognitive ability, including learning and memory deficits in presymptomatic gene carriers may be present compared to their noncarrier relatives.

Huntington disease is a progressive disorder for which there is no cure, so the individual will die in anything from 10 to 20 years from onset of movement symptoms. The symptoms of Huntington disease involve involuntary, uncontrollable, jerking movements of the limbs, head and trunk. These movements are called **chorea** (chorea = *dance*) and they disrupt the patient's normal daily existence and dominate their every purposeful movement. These patients also suffer an ataxia, an eventual loss of speech (a **dysarthria** = imperfect articulation of speech), and behavioural changes, including depression, apathy and irritability (Hofmann 1999). There is often an intellectual decline associated with the disorder. Some develop a degree of dementia and others have schizophrenic-like psychoses, with excitable outbursts, to complicate the picture. The psychotic symptoms are suspected to be caused by the degeneration of the dorsal part of the caudate nucleus (Hofmann 1999).

The overriding cause of this disorder is undoubtedly a genetic error that has been mapped to **chromosome 4**, specifically **4p16.3** (Figure 11.6). This is an autosomal dominant gene and an affected parent has a 50% chance of passing the mutated gene to any of their offspring. The normal gene codes for a protein named **huntingtin** and patients with Huntington disease produce both the normal and abnormal forms of the protein.

See page 79
The gene mutation is called a **trinucleotide repeat**, where the repeated bases are **CAG** (**cytosine–adenine–guanine**). The normal gene changes by duplicating this trinucleotide base many times and the number of repeats present determines the onset or not of symptoms: those with fewer than 30 repeats have no symptoms, but the presence of more than 38 repeats causes symptoms of the disease. If the gene is passed to the offspring from the mother, the number of repeats tends to be copied faithfully: given a mother

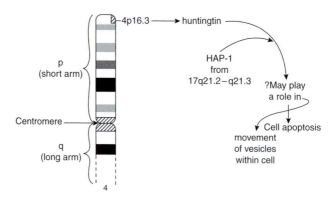

FIGURE 11.6 The 4th chromosome with the huntingtin gene at 4p16.3. Huntingtin binds with huntingtin-associated protein-1 (HAP-1) from chromosome 17.

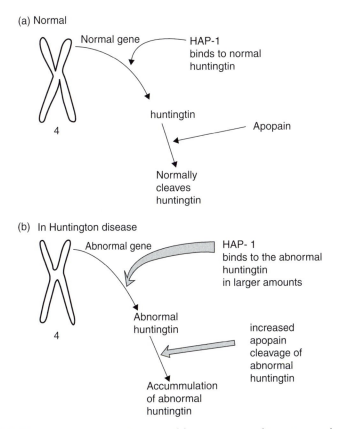

(a) Normal

Normal gene

HAP-1
binds to normal
huntingtin

huntingtin

Apopain

4

Normally
cleaves
huntingtin

(b) In Huntington disease

Abnormal gene

HAP- 1
binds to the abnormal
huntingtin
in larger amounts

Abnormal
huntingtin

4

increased
apopain
cleavage of
abnormal
huntingtin

Accummulation
of abnormal
huntingtin

FIGURE 11.7 Huntingtin protein in normal brain tissue and Huntington disease.

with, say, 30 repeats, the offspring will receive 30 repeats. But if the mutant gene is passed to the offspring from the father (which is more common), variation can occur in the number of repeats the offspring receives. The greater the number of repeats, the earlier the age of onset of symptoms (see **anticipation**).

See page 81

CAG codes for the amino acid **glutamine** and multiple repeats of CAG result in a huntingtin protein with a long glutamine 'tail'. How this affects the function of huntingtin is not yet known since the exact function of the normal protein is not fully understood. However, some clues are emerging as to how the mutant form of this protein can cause the disease (Figure 11.7).

Normal huntingtin. It is known that the normal huntingtin protein is expressed widely in the brain and is essential for normal brain development. It is found in the cytoplasm of the cell, but not in the nucleus. It binds to another protein call **huntingtin-associated protein-1 (HAP-1)**. The normal huntingtin may be a protein that inhibits neuronal cell **apoptosis**, or programmed cell death. If this were the case, the presence of normal huntingtin would prevent the loss of neurons by the natural destruction of cells. HAP-1 could be an inhibitor of huntingtin, blocking its normal role and allowing apoptosis to occur. Huntingtin is also considered to be involved somehow in the normal structure or function of microtubules), which are essential for the role of axonal transportation and the cell's cytoskeleton.

Huntingtin mutation. The addition of CAG repeats to the gene, thus forming a glutamate 'tail' on the molecule, causes the binding of much more HAP-1 than normal to huntingtin. HAP-1 then increases its inhibitory role on huntingtin, possibly allowing increased apoptosis with resultant cell losses. **Apopain** is a proteolytic enzyme (an enzyme for breaking down proteins), and this enzyme splits the normal huntingtin protein, a process that is increased with the mutant abnormal huntingtin protein. The result is the accumulation of huntingtin fragments, some of which form clumps *inside* the nucleus (remember that normal huntingtin is found in the cytoplasm only). These clumps within the nucleus are called **neuronal intranuclear inclusions** (**NII**) and they contain huntingtin fragments together with another protein called **ubiquitin**. Ubiquitin is a universal protein found throughout nature (the name comes from *ubiquitous*) and it appears to join with other proteins when those proteins are to be destroyed. It is one of the proteins found in the core of Lewy bodies. Experiments have suggested that the abnormal huntingtin fragments enter the nucleus and cause damage there. The presence of ubiquitin seems to slow that process down and encourages the formation of NII as a means of tying up the harmful huntingtin fragments to help to prevent the damage (Quarrell 1999). However, this process is probably only a delaying tactic as the damage continues slowly and the loss of normal huntingtin from the cytoplasm continues to prevent normal cytoskeletal production and function.

See page 226

This gives two molecular bases for the possible effects we see in this disease (Figure 11.7):

- increased inhibition of huntingtin by HAP-1, allowing increased apoptosis;
- increased cleavage of huntingtin by apopain, resulting in a loss of the cytoskeletal function of huntingtin and damage to the nucleus.

The mitochondrial DNA may also be implicated in HD. An 11-fold increase in mitochondrial DNA deletions was found in the temporal lobes, and a 5-fold increase in the frontal lobes, of HD patients when compared to controls. This may be due to free radical damage to the DNA in HD patients, but it is uncertain what bearing this has on the disease pathology. The changes seen in the biochemistry are also unexplained at present. A 50% reduction in serotonin and muscarinic receptors is found in the caudate nucleus, but whether that is a cause of some symptoms or simply a measure of caudate nucleus cell losses is not clear.

Treatment of Huntington disease is not really an option at present. There is no cure and there is little in the way of drug treatment to improve the quality of life. **Tetrabenazine** can help to control the abnormal movements. This drug reduces dopamine synthesis in doperminergic neurons, but it has caused some patients to develop depression as a side-effect. Sensitive nursing care, both in the patient's home at first and later in hospital, is the mainstay of effective management of this disorder.

Genetic testing has become available for families with Huntington disease, to see who in the family carries the gene and who does not. However, the implications of this are enormous, given the 100% penetrance of the gene (i.e. if present, the gene will definitely cause the disease). Any individual learning that they carry the gene will know that they will suffer and die from this disease. Worse still, they may have to live with the thought that they might have passed it on to their children. The only advantage would be for those who know they carry the gene and who are without children, as they would then have the ability to make a conscious decision whether or not to have children. It may be worth considering that sometimes not knowing is the better choice to take.

See page 76

Wilson's disease and Harvey's disease

Dr S. A. Wilson (1878–1937) described a familial lenticular degeneration in 1912 (Wilson 1912). Wilson's disease, as it was later called, is an autosomal recessive disorder of copper metabolism (Figure 11.8). The genetic problem

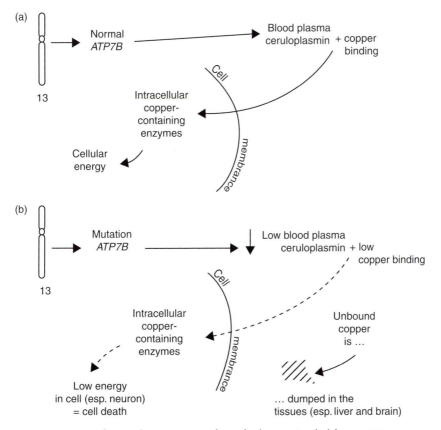

FIGURE 11.8 Wilson's disease. Normal ceruloplasmin (coded by *ATP7B* gene on chromosome 13) binds copper in the plasma and assists its movement into the cell. Here it is used by the enzymes that generate cellular energy. In Wilson's disease, gene error (mutation) causes low ceruloplasmin, and copper cannot enter the cell. The cell runs low on energy and the spare copper accumulates in the tissues, mostly the liver and the brain.

is one of several possible mutations of the gene *ATP7B*, which is localised to 13q14.3–q21.1. The genetic error causes a reduction in the amount of a blood plasma component called **ceruloplasmin**. Ceruloplasmin is normally synthesised in the **Golgi apparatus**, a structure within the cytoplasm that packages, modifies and transports cellular products to a storage site within the cell or out of the cell altogether. Ceruloplasmin is involved in the transportation of copper into the cells, where it becomes integrated into copper-containing enzymes such as **cytochrome oxidase**. Cytochromes are proteins involved in the energy-producing chain found on the inner mitochondrial membrane (Adds *et al.* 1996). Cytochrome oxidase enzyme is usually found to be in a low state of activity in Wilson's disease, causing a failure in energy production. Copper that cannot enter the cells builds up in the body and is deposited in various tissues, notably the liver, the brain and the eyes. The result is both neurological deficits and liver **cirrhosis** (i.e. hepatic **necrosis**, the death of liver cells). The damage in the brain occurs mostly to the **lenticular nuclei** (a combination of the putamen with the globus pallidus) and some degree of cerebral dementia can occur. Symptoms include severe involuntary movements at a young age (10–25 years), leading to progressive mental deterioration. Liver failure occurs later in the course of the disease. Unlike brain cells, liver cells are able to regenerate to a certain extent, so the effects of liver involvement are not felt until the disease is more advanced. **Hypercalciuria**, excessive calcium in the urine, is seen in many cases of Wilson's disease and is sometimes found early, before the neurological symptoms occur. It is probable that the reabsorption mechanism of calcium from the renal tubule is in some way disturbed. Excessive renal calcium can cause stones (or **renal calculi**) to form in the kidneys.

Treatment of Wilson's disease is based on the drug **penicillamine**, which promotes the elimination of copper from the body. If it is treated early enough, all further progress of the disease can be halted. The problem remains, however, that the damage already done cannot be repaired.

History: The strange case of Harvey's disease

During training as a psychiatric student nurse between 1965 and 1968 at Bexley Hospital, Kent (now closed and redeveloped), the author was allocated to a ward called East Hospital. On arrival at this ward, the author was instructed to read a certain set of notes belonging to a patient who was on the ward at that time. The patient was suffering a form of genetically inherited subcortical dementia, which was only present in that one family. The disease had already killed everyone else in his family and our patient was the last family member to die. On his death, the disease would never be seen again as the gene was not passed on to any other generation, nor found in any other family. This was then a very rare example of a genetic disorder becoming extinct.

The symptoms were similar to those of Parkinson's disease or Wilson's disease, but the copper metabolism was normal. He had lost his speech; his mouth was held open and was filled with a handkerchief. He had a very unsteady stiff gait, walking almost on tiptoes, and falling over frequently due to the imbalance caused when the legs could not keep up with the top half of the body.

On the ward his condition was named after him with the family name of Harvey. However, the author has never been able to find any publication concerning this now extinct condition. Surely it must have occurred to a doctor at that time, given the uniqueness of the case, that publication of a paper describing the disease would be useful. Apparently not, and this very brief history, based as it is on the author's memory of the events, may be the only published record of this genetic disease that killed an entire family.

Key points

The basal ganglia

- The subcortical dementias, essentially degeneration of the basal ganglia, are often associated with depression and psychoses.
- The basal ganglia form part of a loop that regulates motor function. This loop consists of the frontal cortex, the corpus striatum, the globus pallidus, the substantia nigra pars reticulum, the thalamus and back to the frontal lobe.

Parkinson's disease

- Muscle rigidity and tremor of the limbs are the classic signs of Parkinson's disease.
- The symptoms of Parkinson's disease are caused by a gradual loss of the substantia nigra cells. Muscle tone therefore increases unopposed.
- The nigrostriatal pathway develops very low dopamine levels, below a threshold of 80% loss of dopamine, before symptoms of the disease occur.
- The low dopamine level causes inhibition of the thalamic role in modifying control of movement by the frontal lobe.
- It is probable that both genetic and environmental factors are involved in the cause of this disease.
- Levodopa replaces dopamine in the nigrostriatal pathway and thus improves the quality of life. Long-term problems of levodopa have largely been overcome.

Huntington disease

- Huntington disease is an autosomal dominant inherited disorder characterised by a deterioration of the corpus striatum caused by a mutation in a gene on chromosome 4.

- The main signs of Huntington disease are involuntary jerky movements called chorea, speech loss and intellectual decline.
- The gene mutation is a trinucleotide repeat of the bases CAG (cytosine–adenine–guanine) that causes a glutamine tail repeat sequence on the normal huntingtin protein.
- Accumulations of abnormal huntingtin protein fragments in the neuron nucleus and loss of normal huntingtin from the cytoplasm probably cause the cellular degeneration.

Wilson's disease

- Wilson's disease is a familial lenticular degeneration caused by an autosomal recessive gene that results in disorder of copper metabolism.
- The gene is *ATP7B* at 13q14.3–q21.1. Mutations cause a reduction in the amount ceruloplasmin in blood. This disturbs copper transport into neurons. Energy-producing enzymes that use copper fail to function.
- The result is both neurological deficits, caused by damage to the lenticular nuclei, and liver cirrhosis.
- Treatment of Wilson's disease is with the drug penicillamine, which promotes the elimination of copper from the body.

Harvey's disease

- Harvey's disease may have been a very rare example of a familial genetic basal ganglia degenerative disorder that became extinct in the 1960s when the last affected member of the family died.

References

Adds J., Larkcon E. and Miller R. (1996) *Cell Biology and Genetics*. Nelson, Walton-on-Thames.

Aird T. (2000) Functional anatomy of the basal ganglia. *Journal of Neuroscience Nursing*, **32** (5): 250–253.

Bear M. F., Connors B. W. and Paradiso M. A. (1996) *Neuroscience, Exploring the Brain*. Williams and Wilkins, Baltimore.

Borrell E. (2000) Hypokinetic movement disorders. *Journal of Neuroscience Nursing*, **32** (5): 254–255.

Carlson N. (2001) *Physiology of Behavior*. Allyn and Bacon, Boston.

Crabb L. (2001) Sleep disorders in Parkinson's disease: the nursing role. *British Journal of Nursing*, **10** (1): 42–47.

Gray P. and Hildebrand K. (2000) Fall risk factors in Parkinson's disease. *Journal of Neuroscience Nursing*, **32** (4): 222–228.

Herndon C. M., Young K., Herndon A. D. and Dole E. J. (2000) Parkinson's disease revisited. *Journal of Neuroscience Nursing*, **32** (4): 216–221.

Hofmann N. (1999) Understanding the neuropsychiatric symptoms of Huntington's disease. *Journal of Neuroscience Nursing*, **31** (5): 309–313.

Kaplan H. I. and Sadock B. J. (1996) *Concise Textbook of Clinical Psychiatry*. Williams and Wilkins, Baltimore.

Nowak R. (2000) Early warning for Parkinson's. *New Scientist*, **168** (2266): 14.

Quarrell O. (1999) *Huntington's Disease, The Facts*. Oxford University Press, Oxford.

Roberts G. W., Leigh P. N. and Weinberger D. R. (1993) *Neuropsychiatric Disorders*. Wolfe, London.

Wilson S. A. K. (1912) Progressive lenticular degeneration: a familial nervous disease associated with cirrhosis of the liver. *Brain* **34**: 295–507.

Chapter 12

The ageing brain and dementia

- The ageing brain
- The hippocampus and memory
- The dementias
- Alzheimer disease
- The molecular neurobiology of Alzheimer disease
- Dementia with cortical Lewy bodies
- Pick's disease
- The drugs used in dementia
- Key points

The ageing brain

Like all organs, the brain changes as a result of the ageing process (Figure 12.1), but the functions of the brain can be retained virtually untouched to extreme late age in many people. This shows the remarkable compensation the brain is able to undergo to make good the deterioration, and demonstrates that dementia is not inevitable, nor is it caused by ageing.

Age-related neuron losses vary not only between individuals but also between different parts of the brain in the same individual. Naturally occurring neuron loss can begin as early as 21 years of age, but is likely to increase after 60 years of age. In some persons, the total losses of neurons could be as much as 40% – the equivalent of just less than half the brain lost – and yet they can retain good cerebral activity. A very good example of excellent cerebral function in late age is the remarkable English composer Havergal

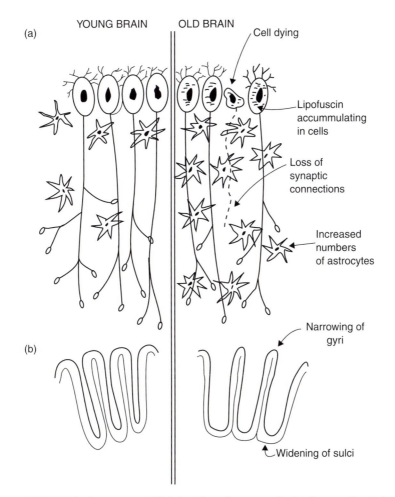

FIGURE 12.1 The brain gets old. (a). Left is the young brain, but on the right the brain shows cell losses with corresponding synaptic losses, increased astrocytes and lipofuscin deposits in the neurons. (b). Narrowing of the gyri and widening of the sulci is a gross anatomical change in the elderly brain.

Brian, who wrote *twenty symphonies* between the ages of 80 and 92 years – an amazing feat of late-age brain activity.

It was thought for many years that neurons were a type of cell that was incapable of replication after birth, so that losses could not be replaced. However, humans are now known to be capable of neuronal replication to a limited extent throughout life, especially in certain brain regions, and this neuron replacement may account for at least part of the retention of good mental function during the normal ageing process. Neuron losses are attributed to reduced blood flow to the brain caused by age-related changes in the arteries that supply the head. Neurons are oxygen-sensitive and will deteriorate and finally die when faced with a decline in the oxygen supply. Each neuron can have thousands of synaptic connections, so one neuron lost can account for thousands of lost synapses. Synapses are vital for memory

See page 244 and learning. The neocortex loses glutamate synapses from around the age of 20 onwards, with about 20% lost by the age of 70 years. Some 40% or so of the glutamate synapses could be lost from the hippocampus with age.

Various studies have demonstrated that dementia is more prevalent among those with the lowest levels of education and least common in groups with higher education, suggesting that brain deterioration is slower in people who undertake intellectual pursuits (Katzman and Kawas 1998). So, as in the case of Havergal Brian, it seems that active use of the brain into old age is most beneficial; a definite case of 'use it, or lose it'? Cognitively challenging careers may add to this decrease in the risk of dementia, as may mental stimulation of children from an early age, possibly causing increased synaptic formation. The effect may also be linked with the blood flow changes associated with brain function; stimulated areas of the brain use and receive more blood and therefore keep the brain active until a late age. Sustaining good cerebral blood and oxygen flow reduces neuronal losses and improves the brain's ability to compensate for those losses that do occur.

Neuronal losses are part of the reason for the brain's loss of protein in old age. About 15% of the protein in the brain is lost between the ages of 35 and 70 years and this is partly responsible for the reduction of brain weight with age, from about 1400 grams in a male aged 20 down to 1200 grams in the same male aged 80. In contrast, both the volume of extracellular water and the number of astrocytes in the brain *increase* with age and the ventricles within the brain enlarge. The cerebral cortex shrinks and shows a widening *See page 3* of the **sulci** and a narrowing of the **gyri**, with atrophy of the frontal lobes predominating. **Lipofuscin**, an age-related pigment based on lipid, is deposited inside the ageing cells, more so in the brain than anywhere else. The amount varies in different parts of the brain. The function, if any, of lipofuscin is unknown and whether it has any effect on the cell to promote ageing is unclear. The brain's chemistry also changes with age; noradrenaline and dopamine levels slowly decline in some parts and this has been linked to depression in some elderly persons.

The hippocampus and memory

The hippocampus is situated within the hippocampal fissure, close to the parahippocampal gyrus, part of the temporal lobes on both sides (see Chapter 1 and Figures 1.4, 7.1 and 8.2) (Blows 2000). This area is sometimes called the **hippocampal complex** or **hippocampal formation**, because several structures occur close together and have many interconnections with each other. The components of the complex are:

See page 165
- **dentate gyrus**, the innermost cell layer of the hippocampus;
- **Ammon's horn** (see Figure 8.2), another part of the hippocampus, consisting also of a layer of neurons that can be subdivided into four areas, **CA1**, **CA2**, **CA3** and **CA4** (where CA means *cornu Ammonis*, or 'Ammon's horn') (Figure 12.2);

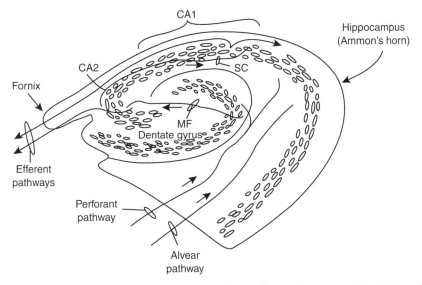

FIGURE 12.2 The hippocampus. Ammon's horn cells are shown as CA1, CA2 and CA3. MF is the mossy fibre pathway, SC is the Schaffer collateral pathway.

- **subiculum**, also included in the hippocampus by some authors (e.g. Haines 1995) (Figure 8.2); *See page 165*
- **entorhinal cortex**, which lies between the subiculum and the perirhinal cortex (Figure 8.2); *See page 165*
- **perirhinal cortex**, which lies between the entorhinal cortex and the parahippocampal cortex (Figure 8.2);
- **parahippocampal cortex**, the outermost component of the complex (Figures 7.1, 8.2). *See page 165*

The connections between these areas and with other parts of the brain are:

- afferent (incoming) pathways into the entorhinal cortex from the **cingulum**;
- afferent pathways into the entorhinal cortex from the major sensory association areas of the cortex, e.g. visual, auditory, **somatosensory** (i.e. from the body) and **gustatory** (taste) areas;
- **perforant pathway**, from the entorhinal cortex to Ammon's horn and dentate gyrus (Figure 12.2);
- **alvear pathway**, from the entorhinal cortex to Ammon's horn (Figure 12.2);
- **mossy fibre pathway**, from the dentate gyrus to CA3 of Ammon's horn (Figure 12.2);
- **Schaffer collateral pathway**, from CA3 to CA1 of Ammon's horn (Figure 12.2);
- efferent (outgoing) pathways via the **fornix** (the main axonal pathways leaving the hippocampus) to areas of the frontal cortex, thalamus and the hypothalamus (especially the **mammillary bodies**) (Figure 12.2).

See page 8
The hippocampus has several important roles. These include maintaining the **short-term memory** (which is closely related to learning) and influencing thinking through connections with the frontal cortex. It also has a part *See page 148* to play in emotions, especially the regulation of **aggression**. It is closely linked to the adrenal hormone cortisol, regulating cortisol release via the hypothalamus and pituitary gland pathway. Cortisol is the hormone that is increased during stress, so the hippocampus is also part of the brain's normal *See page 140* stress response.

How memory works

There are several ways of classifying memory, one way being the division into **long-term memory** and **short-term memory**, i.e. the difference between remembering events which took place 20 years ago and events that happened 20 minutes ago. Another way is the division into **explicit memory** and **implicit memory**, i.e. the difference between memory that comes with *conscious thought* – for example, trying to remember Aunt Edith's telephone number – and *automatic* or *subconscious* memory such as finding the way from your bedroom to the bathroom at home. These classifications are roughly correlated in that long-term memory is broadly implicit, while short-term memory is more likely to be explicit. The term 'commit to memory' implies a shift of memorised facts or skills from explicit to implicit memory; that is, making the memory automatic or long-term. This is achieved by *rehearsal* of the facts or skill, often many times, in much the same way as an actor memorises the lines of a play, a pianist prepares for a concert or a tennis player practises for a match. There is no substitute for the rehearsal of facts; it is crucial for all implicit (or long-term) memory activities, such as taking examinations. It is the basis of the *learning process*, an essential ingredient of success for all aspiring actors, pianists and tennis stars, as well as those hoping to pass examinations.

At a biochemical level, the processes of memory have not been so easy to understand. However, there is now an established and growing volume of evidence to suggest that memory is the result of neurons producing and maintaining a **long-term potentiation** (LTP) (Bear *et al.* 1996). This is a permanent (or at least semipermanent) change in the synapse that occurs in the hippocampus and other parts of the brain as a result of activation by a specific excitatory action potential (or stimulus). The formation of this change, a state of heightened stimulation in the synaptic membrane that occurs each time a specific impulse arrives, requires the function of glutamate acting on *See page 49* NMDA receptors and the presence of calcium. A similar, but depressive (inhibitory), effect on the synapse is called **long-term depression** (LTD, not to be confused with the disorder). Between them, LTP and LTD may provide the synaptic mechanism for **declarative memory**, i.e. memory for facts and events. But these changes are temporary (short-term memory); for a memory to become a long-term memory requires further molecular manipulation. It is a complex process, but a brief and simplified outline is given here because the end product is important in the understanding of what happens in dementia.

After the formation of LTP or LTD at the synapse, certain proteins have had a phosphate group added to them (a process called **phosphorylation**). After a period of time (anything from days to months) the phosphate group will be removed and the protein will be degraded and replaced by a non-phosphorylated version. If this happens, the LTP or LTD will have been lost (along with the memory). To retain the memory in the long term, the phosphorylated protein must be replaced by a permanent version of the protein. This permanent protein replacement appears to be involved in the conversion of short-term memory to long-term memory. Repeated recreation of the original LTP or LTD at the synapse reinforces this replacement of proteins to the permanent form, just as repeated exposure to the same information (i.e. the same stimuli) reinforces learning. The formation of the permanent proteins finally leads to the *creation of new synapses*. These new synapses forming in the brain are known to occur as a result of learning. It becomes a sobering thought when we consider that children go to school to have new synapses formed in their brains! Yet this highlights a fundamental point about the processes of learning and memory. The brains that are best suited to learning and memory are the brains of children. All the anatomy of the brain is in place at birth, but the nervous system is far from mature at that point. The development of the nervous system involves the formation of new synaptic connections, and this continues throughout childhood until puberty, so learning is a major part of this process. The bulk of synaptic formation occurs during the childhood years and this is exactly the time when the brain is best suited to forming the permanent proteins and synapses needed for memory. Adult brains are somewhat more resistant to this kind of change, although of course learning does take place in the mature brain.

The relevance of all this to dementia is that forgetting (and long-term memory loss is a major feature of dementia) can be seen as a loss of the permanent synapses as neurons die. A single neuron can have thousands of synapses, so the loss of key neurons in the brain is likely to interfere with memory significantly. What education in childhood has created, dementia can destroy; but the more advanced the education (and therefore good synaptic formations) the harder it becomes for this destruction to take place.

Memory is not found in one place in the brain; many areas serve to store information which can be retrieved when required, so-called **working memory**. However, the conscious working memory is primarily the role of the frontal lobes, the prefrontal cortex particularly. Here, memory and thought work together on matters that concern us at any particular moment. The prefrontal cortex is vital for the memory needed for spatial tasks, remembering objects, self-ordered tasks and analytical reasoning (Beardsley 1997). Input into this frontal lobe activity is via the hippocampus. With the retrieval of short-term memory at its disposal, and with the influence it has on thinking and emotions, the hippocampus is a powerful tool in the processing of thought. It is not surprising that problems arising with the hippocampus seriously disrupt not only memory, but also the whole ability to think properly.

Declarative memory is divided into **semantic memory**, i.e. the raw facts and figures, and **episodic memory**, the context in which these facts and figures occur. For example:

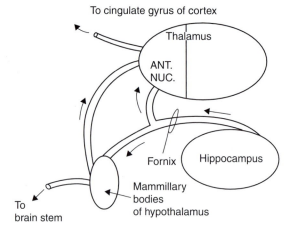

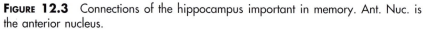

FIGURE 12.3 Connections of the hippocampus important in memory. Ant. Nuc. is the anterior nucleus.

- **semantic** = 9 is a number; **episodic** = 9 is the ninth numerate in a set sequence of numerates that start at 1.
- **semantic** = fish have gills; **episodic** = gills are part of a system by which animal life extracts oxygen from its environments.

Hippocampal memory appears to be the result of LTPs in CA1, and to a lesser extent in CA3 of Ammon's horn. Damage to these cell layers appears to impair episodic memory and cause **anterograde amnesia** (i.e. memory loss occurring after some form of brain injury). To lose *all* declarative memory requires lesions of the brain that involve both the limbic areas of the medial temporal lobe and the hippocampus. In fact, lesions anywhere, from the hippocampus through the fornix to the mammillary bodies and anterior thalamus, can disrupt memory. It would appear that this circuit is critical in the formation and recall of memories (Figure 12.3).

The dementias

Dementia means 'loss of mind' and occurs in various forms depending on both the cause and its effects. Dementia can be caused by extensive brain damage from a head injury, **cerebral infections** or **cerebral infarctions**, or compression of the brain from a **space-occupying lesion** (**SOL**) or from a biochemical imbalance. Vascular disease, reducing the arterial blood supply to the brain with increasing age (**cerebral ischaemia**), causes about 15–25% of dementia cases. Starved of blood, the oxygen-sensitive neurons die and may be replaced with scar tissue. Trauma (head injury) accounts for only about 3% of dementias. The different types of dementia include:

- **attentional dementia** with some loss of arousal of the conscious mind;
- **intentional dementia** with loss of vigilance;
- **cognitive dementia** with a loss of remote memory;

- **amnestic dementia** with a loss of recent memory;
- **multi-infarct dementia**, caused by a number of minor strokes;
- **Binswanger dementia**, due to **hypertension** (high blood pressure), which causes vascular disease in the brain and neuronal white matter destruction;
- **dementia with cortical Lewy bodies** (**DCLB**) (about 10% of dementias); *See page 254*
- **Pick's disease**, dementia with characteristic cortical Pick bodies; *See page 254*
- **Alzheimer disease** (**AD**), a form of dementia with characteristic brain changes found at post mortem (about 45% of dementias).

Alzheimer disease (AD)

In Alzheimer disease (AD), two main forms of the disease are recognised: an early-age onset (before 65 years) showing a family history of inherited genetic origin (i.e. **familial Alzheimer disease, FAD**) and a late-age onset (after 65 years) of less genetic and more sporadic origin. This disorder has been, and still is, the subject of intensive research for several reasons. First, the pathology of AD is related to other brain-destructive disorders like Parkinson disease and Huntington disease. Advances in the understanding of one of these disorders may provide useful insights into the others. Second, there is a very interesting link between AD and **Down syndrome**. *See page 83* Third, the devastation caused by this disease, both to the patient and to the family, is catastrophic, as it usually occurs at a time of life when an ageing partner is ill-equipped to care for a demented spouse. It reduces formerly highly intelligent people to a pitiful state, with no hope of recovery. The fear that any of us could end our days in this manner drives research forward in an attempt to prevent the tragedy. Dementia causes erosion of personality; relatives say that the patient is nothing like their former self. Mood changes with emotional blunting occur, with abnormal and inappropriate behaviour, especially restless wandering at any time of the day or night. People with dementia develop a state of self-neglect and need everything done for them. One important form of self-neglect is that these people may suffer from a lack of adequate nutrition. Several factors combine to cause this, including memory losses (e.g. when to eat, how to prepare food), inadequate supervision by family carers or hospital staff, poor oral hygiene and constipation. Nurses can improve the person's overall state of health by effective interventions to maintain a healthy mouth and bowels, and by ensuring that nutritious meals are eaten by the patient daily (Biernacki and Barratt 2001).

Memory loss and confusion are perhaps the problems for which this disorder is best known. **Amnesia** (memory loss) at first is primarily short-term: the patient can, say, remember where they were during the war, but cannot remember what they had for breakfast. **Confusion** is not uncommon in the elderly in any case and is often *acute*, i.e. relatively short-lived and caused by a physical problem which may be easily correctable, such as constipation, sleep loss, fever or a drug side-effect. Other, more difficult conditions which can cause confusion, especially in the elderly, are cardiac, renal or liver failure; blood glucose instability in diabetes; other endocrine and metabolic disorders, such as acidosis, epilepsy, vitamin deficiencies, malnutrition or dehydration, postanaesthetic or other drug withdrawal, head injury, brain tumours, or stress. Confusion which is persistent, after all the physical causes have been eliminated, may be a sign of dementia.

Preserving cognitive and functional abilities in the Alzheimer's disease patient is central to the role of the nurse (Maier-Lorentz 2000b). Nursing interventions can be most valuable in overcoming the problems of failing memory, behavioural difficulties (e.g. wandering), language problems (e.g. errors in the language), impaired **visuospatial function** (e.g. confusion in an unfamiliar environment), sleep disturbance and psychotic episodes (notably depression, delusions and hallucinations) (Maier-Lorentz 2000a,b).

The molecular neurobiology of Alzheimer disease

Alzheimer was a German psychiatrist who in 1907 described a dementia with two specific changes found in the brain after death. These changes were the presence of *extracellular* **plaques** and *intracellular* **neurofibrillary tangles (NFT)** and these became the hallmarks of this disease, i.e. they were diagnostic for Alzheimer disease at post mortem. Alzheimer disease is a progressive deterioration of brain function associated with neuronal losses. Before the age of 65 about 1% of the population are sufferers and by the age of 85 the figure is 10% of the population. The devastating effects of the disease on the individual and their family, together with a proportional increase in the elderly population resulting in greater numbers of people suffering from the disease, makes it a major mental health problem. After years of difficulties, much progress has now been achieved in understanding the pathology of Alzheimer disease and it is expected that research will continue to make strides towards prevention of its worst effects.

The plaques

The plaques described by Alzheimer are made from the central core of an abnormal amyloid protein called **Aβ42** (beta-amyloid, 42 amino acids long). Normally Aβ42 exists in very small quantities in the brain, but it accumulates in large amounts in Alzheimer disease, hence the abnormality.

The biology of amyloid protein is still largely unknown and is the subject of intense research. What is known is that a large gene on chromosome 21 called the *APP* gene (Figure 12.4) codes for the normal protein called **APP (amyloid β precursor protein)**. Normal amyloid protein (APP) is still partly a mystery in the brain, its functions not being fully understood. It may be a protease inhibitor (i.e. blocking the enzymes that break down other proteins), it could have a role in cell growth or adhesion (i.e. maintaining the cell in its correct place) or it may act as a cell surface receptor. Better known is the role of the **Aβ domain** (part of APP), which is essential for the axonal transport of APP to the synapse (see Figure 2.2). Here, at the synapse, APP appears to be very important for thought processing and memory. In the cell body, prior to axonal transportation, APP is found inside the **endoplasmic reticulum (ER)** of the neuron where it is normally cloven (or cut) into the

See page 24

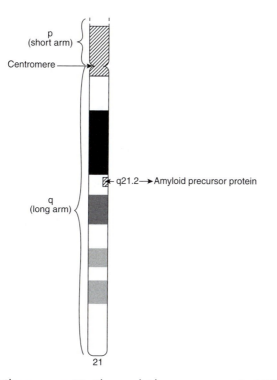

FIGURE 12.4 Chromosome 21. The amyloid precursor protein (*APP*) gene is at 21q21.2.

Aβ40 form (40 amino acids long, i.e. a shorter chain version than the abnormal **Aβ42**) (Figure 12.5). Cleavage of APP into Aβ40 is thought to involve two further proteins, **presenilin 1 (PS1)** and **presenilin 2 (PS2)**, the genes for coding these proteins being on chromosome 14 and chromosome 1, respectively. More is known about PS1 than about PS2. PS1 attaches across the ER membrane, influencing APP cleavage within the ER. PS2 may bind to APP and affect its cleavage by this means. One further gene involved is the ***ERAB* gene** on chromosome X, coding for the **ERAB protein (endoplasmic reticulum-associated binding protein)**. This protein, of unknown function, attaches itself normally to the outside of the ER membrane. It appears to be important in the abnormal mechanism that leads to extracellular plaque formation in AD.

In **Familiar Alzheimer disease (FAD)**, mutations within the *APP* (**chromosome 21**), *PS-1* (**chromosome 14**), *PS-2* (**chromosome 1**) and *ERAB* (**chromosome X**) genes cause errors in the proteins that these genes code for, leading to mistakes in the way these proteins function. Mutations are abnormal changes in the DNA (deoxyribosenucleic acid) code within the chromosome, thus creating abnormal proteins. In the case of the *APP* gene the mutation results in excessive APP protein, while mutations in the *PS-1* and *PS-2* genes cause errors in the cleavage of APP from the normal Aβ40 form to the abnormal Aβ42 form. The combination of all three mutations results in a large accumulation within the ER of the neuron of the Aβ42

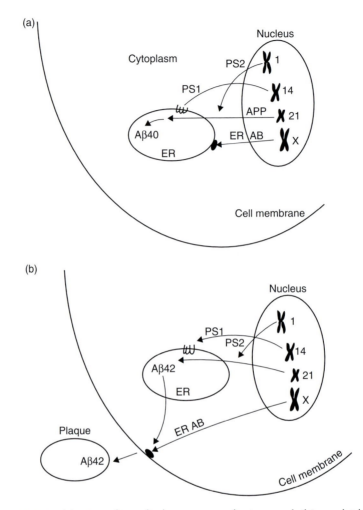

Figure 12.5 (a) Normal amyloid protein production, and (b) amyloid plaque formation outside the cell in Alzheimer disease. ER is the endoplasmic reticulum.

protein. Somehow this Aβ42 must find its way out of the neuron to become extracellular plaques. Here, mutations of the *ERAB* gene (chromosome X) may be the answer, since faulty ERAB protein no longer locates to the ER but finds a new site of accumulation inside the perimeter cell membrane, binding Aβ42 at the same time. This shift of site for ERAB protein may well be the transport mechanism for Aβ42 to get from the ER to outside the cell (Figure 12.5). Once accumulated between the neurons, Aβ42 allows for the development of abnormal glial cell production and accumulation (a **gliosis**, mostly of **astrocytes**).

The neurofibrillary tangles

The tangles inside the neurons described by Alzheimer are made from an abnormal form of **tau protein**. Normal tau protein binds to the protein

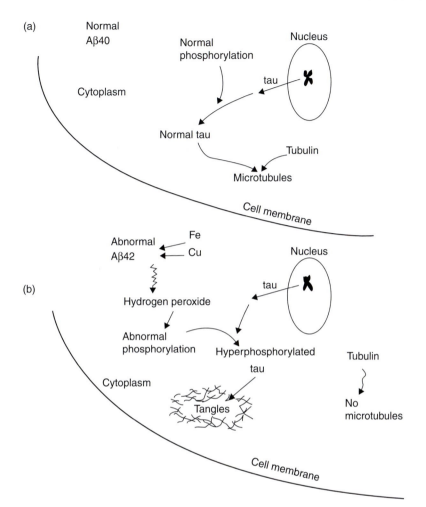

(a)

Normal
Aβ40

Normal
phosphorylation

Nucleus

Cytoplasm

tau

Normal tau

Tubulin

Microtubules

Cell membrane

(b)

Abnormal
Aβ42

Fe

Cu

Nucleus

Hydrogen peroxide

tau

Abnormal
phosphorylation

Hyperphosphorylated
tau

Tubulin

Cytoplasm

Tangles

No
microtubules

Cell membrane

FIGURE 12.6 (a) Normal tau synthesis and (b) abnormal tau tangles in Alzheimer disease. Fe and Cu are the chemical symbols for iron and copper, respectively.

tubulin, the main component of the cell microtubules, and tau is essential for the stabilisation of the cell cytoskeleton. Microtubules are also vital for functions such as axonal transport and abnormal tau may be partly responsible for disruption of this process. The abnormal form of tau accumulates as tangles (Figure 12.6).

See page 24
See page 24

The process by which this happens is both complex and not yet fully worked out. In AD, the neurons of the temporal and frontal lobes, and also of the hippocampus, lose up to 70% of a particular enzyme called **choline acetyltransferase (ChAT).** This enzyme loss causes a reduction in the choline content of these cells. The result is an adverse affect on APP cleavage, leading to an increased amount of Aβ protein inside the cell. These higher levels of Aβ protein contribute to a process called **oxidative stress** involving an increase in the production of **reactive oxygen species,** highly reactive chemical agents based on oxygen which damage cellular processes.

A mechanism for this has been identified whereby Aβ protein binds two metals, iron and copper, and in the process these metals donate electrons to oxygen. The negatively charged oxygen then reacts with hydrogen to form **hydrogen peroxide**, a highly reactive and damaging compound. In this case, the damage is disruption of the normal **phosphorylation–dephosphorylation cycle** of proteins in the cell. The phosphorylation (adding of a phosphate to proteins) and dephosphorylation (removal of a phosphate from proteins) is a mechanism for activating or deactivating proteins. The disruption of this process as a result of oxidative stress causes **hyperphosphorylation** of tau (i.e. tau becomes bound with too much phosphate and thus accumulates as tangles). The absence of normal tau causes tubulin to fail in its role of microtubule formation (Figure 12.6).

See page 234

Two other proteins are apparently involved in AD. The first is called **ubiquitin** and attaches to the abnormal tau at a late stage during tangle formation, but its role is unclear. The second is a newly discovered protein called **AMY 117** which forms lesions in the same brain regions as the plaques found in both AD and elderly Down syndrome patients. This protein can occupy up to one-third of the diseased brain in AD and always appears to form together with the beta-amyloid plaques. This has led to speculation that it may be involved in helping to form the beta-amyloid plaques. However, the actual role of this protein in both the normal brain and in the pathology of AD has to be fully worked out (Schmidt *et al.* 1997).

The genetics of AD

See page 247

As noted before, the early-age onset form of the disease (before 65 years) is more often genetically inherited than the late-age onset form (after 65 years). FAD studies often show multiple mutations in three autosomal dominant genes, namely the *APP* (chromosome 21), *PS-1* (chromosome 14) and *PS-2* genes (chromosome 1) (Bentley 1999). In the over-65

See page 249

age group, the genetic evidence is less compelling, but 20–40% of this group show a genetic error on the **ApoE (apolipoprotein E) gene** on **chromosome 19**. Three forms of the ApoE gene have been found in studies of the Northern European population; *ApoE$_\varepsilon$-2* (8% of the population), *ApoE$_\varepsilon$-3* (77% of the population), and *ApoE$_\varepsilon$-4* (15% of the population). It is the *ApoE$_\varepsilon$-4* version that is the mutation that predisposes for AD. *ApoE$_\varepsilon$-4* at one allele results in AD starting in the *late* sixties and seventies age group, while the gene present at both alleles doubles the risk of developing the disease and brings the onset age to the *early* sixties. Mutant ApoE (apolipoprotein E) adds to the accumulation of Aβ42 in plaque formation.

See page 210

Mitochondrial DNA may also have a role to play in some dementias, notably Alzheimer disease (see Figure 10.6). This genetic material, a loop of DNA in the mitochondrion, is always inherited from the maternal line. Alzheimer disease could result from failure of genes that produce **transfer ribonucleic acid (tRNA)** molecules inside the mitochondrion. These would normally be essential for protein synthesis, a process that would be severely disrupted, causing neuronal death, if these genes become faulty. Mitochondrial DNA mutations may play a more important role in the sporadic (i.e. non-inherited) forms of the disease.

Inflammation in AD

New information is emerging suggesting a link between inflammation, the brain's phagocytic cells and Alzheimer disease (Katzman and Kawas 1998). Observations made on patients with diseases such as arthritis have identified that those patients taking steroids have a low incidence of Alzheimer disease. The anti-inflammatory effect of the steroids apparently dampens an immune reaction in the brain caused by the protein beta-amyloid. The phagocytic cells of the brain, called **microglia**, would normally clear away the debris *See page 36* which occurs in the brain. Instead, in AD they appear to produce toxins that cause neuron destruction. From this stems the idea that anti-inflammatory drugs may slow the progress of the disease. Not everyone should take steroids, of course, but other **nonsteroidal anti-inflammatory drugs** (**NSAIDs**) may benefit the Alzheimer patient.

Inflammation is often, but not always, caused by an infectious organism, and some post-mortem brain samples taken from Alzheimer disease patients have revealed the presence of the bacterium *Chlamydia pneumoniae*. This *intracellular* organism was located to the temporal lobes and hippocampus, just the areas affected most by this disease. This does not, of course, prove that the organism is the cause of AD; rather it may increase the risk of developing the disorder. Microglia and astrocytes appear to be the main cells in which this organism survives, and the fact that it lives *inside* the neuron makes it more difficult to treat. It is suspected that persons with the mutant ApoE gene are more susceptible to *Chlamydia pneumoniae* infection.

Diet and AD

High levels of the amino acid **homocysteine** have been found in the blood of AD sufferers and very high levels found in nonsufferers appear to increase their risk of developing the disease (Smith *et al.* 1998). This substance is potentially harmful in large quantities as it known to be toxic to nerve cells. The high level of homocysteine is related to low levels of **vitamin B$_{12}$** (called **cyanocobalamin**) and of **folic acid** (or **folate**) in the circulation, suggesting that there is a lack of these nutrients in the person's diet. Reducing the levels of homocysteine may be achievable by increasing the dietary intake of these vitamins. However, it is not entirely clear whether the high levels of homocysteine are a cause of AD or whether they are perhaps the effect of early AD before any symptoms occur (i.e. when it is **asymptomatic**). Evidence points tentatively more towards the former, but caution is urged before anyone considers taking any vitamin supplements. Excess vitamins can themselves be harmful and a balanced diet would normally provide all the body's needs.

Association of AD with Down syndrome

See page 83

Down syndrome is a trisomy 21 (three chromosomes 21 instead of two). Chromosome 21 is the site of the *APP* gene, which means that Down syndrome sufferers carry three copies of this gene in every cell. Several interesting correlations have been found to link AD with Down syndrome:

- Down syndrome sufferers develop Alzheimer-like dementia at 30+ years and have been found to have multiple, diffuse plaque formation up to 10 years before dementia symptoms arise.
- Elderly (non-Down) patients with AD appear to have had a higher than average number of Down syndrome children earlier in their lives.

Those affected with Down syndrome express five times more APP in the brain than normal owing to the 50% extra APP present. The risk of developing AD is proportional to the amount of APP produced by the three copies of the gene present.

Dementia with cortical Lewy bodies (DCLB)

See page 226

DCLB, or cortical Lewy body disease, accounts for about 10% of all dementias, but about 20% of Alzheimer disease patients also have Lewy bodies (i.e. they have a combination of AD with DCLB, and DCLB may be a variation of AD), and about 2% of the normal elderly population also have Lewy bodies. Lewy bodies are rounded eosinophilic inclusion bodies found in some brain stem nuclei and also in the cerebral cortex. The proposed difference between AD and DCLB is the presence (AD) or absence (DCLB) of neurofibrillary tangles (see Table 12.1) (Roberts *et al.* 1993). The symptoms of DCLB are very much like those of AD but with greater emphasis on motor symptoms such as extrapyramidal tremors. Some additional psychiatric symptoms can occur, as do variations in cognitive ability.

Pick's disease

Pick's dementia was described in 1892, earlier than Alzheimer disease. It is rarer than AD, with 20% of patients showing familial inheritance. Both the genes involved and the cause of the nongenetic cases are unknown. The onset of symptoms mostly occurs at about 50 to 60 years of age, affecting women more than men. The early symptoms show a predominance of social and personality changes rather than memory and intellectual deterioration

TABLE 12.1 The distinction between AD and DCLB

Dementia type	Plaques	Tangles	Lewy bodies
AD	Present	Present	Absent
AD with DCLB	Present	Present	Present
DCLB	Present	Absent	Present

(as in AD). This is due to the neuropathology which is characteristic for this disease. The brain shows a significant atrophy (a loss of superficial neurons) in the anterior *cortical* aspects of the frontal and temporal lobes. The atrophy is rare and less severe in the parietal lobe and extremely rare in the occipital lobe and cerebellum. Astrocytes proliferate in these areas of atrophy, with gliosis (glial cell proliferation) and fibrous tissue deposited.

Neurons in the affected areas become swollen and oval in shape, with an absence of Nissl bodies. In place of the Nissl bodies, abnormal **Pick bodies** fill the cell cytoplasm, pushing the nucleus to one side. Pick bodies are inclusions of neurofilaments similar to neurofibrillary tangles and, like neurofibrillary tangles, they disrupt the cell's internal cytoskeleton. However, the actual neurofibrillary tangles and the plaques seen in AD are both missing in this disease. **Hirano bodies**, another form of intraneuronal inclusion found mostly in the hippocampus, are present in many cases. These are made from deranged cytoskeletal components. Another feature is the extensive loss of myelination within the white matter coming from the affected cortical areas.

The disease causes changes in the personality and social behaviour patterns in the patient during its early stages. The deterioration of social habits may include inappropriate sexual or criminal activities, the patient showing a loss of normal inhibitions and a lack of insight. Changes in mood may be characterised by either apathy or a state of euphoria. As the disease progresses, the patient suffers speech and language difficulties and in the later stages memory and intellect decline.

Variations of this disease have been noted, such as **Pick's disease type II**, where severe gliosis (predominance of glial cells) occurs within the *subcortical* white matter, nuclei, brain stem and parts of the spinal cord. The cortex is less affected, with shrunken cells (not swollen) and mild gliosis.

The drugs used in dementia

Donepezil (**Aricept**) is a reversible acetylcholinesterase inhibitor, used as a treatment of the symptoms of mild to moderate Alzheimer disease. It reduces the rate of cognitive deterioration in about 40% of cases, but has no effect on dementias caused by failure of cerebral circulation. **Rivastigmine** (**Exelon**) is another such inhibitor of acetylcholinesterase. Both of these work by blocking the action of acetylcholinesterase, the enzyme that breaks down acetylcholine, thus increasing the level of acetylcholine in brain circuits devastated by a lack of this neurotransmitter. These drugs can induce unwanted dose-related cholinergic side-effects that include nausea, vomiting, diarrhoea, dizziness, insomnia and rarely **syncopy** (fainting).

Ampakines are another class of drugs that improve memory by a different mechanism (Figure 12.7). They prolong the memory by stimulating glutamate binding to AMPA receptors. Increased AMPA receptor activity then promotes the function of NMDA receptors and thereby establishes improved LTP in the postsynaptic membrane. When they come into clinical practice, ampakines may be the next generation of memory-enhancing drugs to replace the acetylcholinesterase inhibitors (Concar 1997). However, there

See page 244

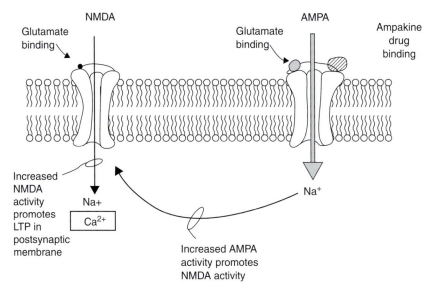

FIGURE 12.7 Ampakine drug action. By binding to AMPA receptors, these drugs increase glutamate activity at that receptor. The increased sodium entry here promotes NMDA receptor activity in the same cell membrane, resulting in a large calcium influx, which boosts memory.

is a down side to memory-boosting drugs. Growing evidence indicates that memory is closely associated with pain, both the memory and the sensation of pain (Day 2002). Boosting memory with drugs may have the adverse affect of increasing pain sensitivity, so everything that hurts normally would hurt even more with these drugs. It is a stark choice for the elderly with dementia: improve your memory but suffer more pain, or live in comfort and memory loss. It may be possible, however, to target the drugs to different areas of the brain, i.e. to the areas that process memory and not to the areas that process pain. In addition, other drugs that block pain-related enzymes in the spine may reduce the sensation of pain in persons taking these drugs (Day 2002).

Key points

The ageing brain

- Naturally occurring neuron loss can begin as early as 21 years of age, but is likely to increase after 60.
- Neuron losses may be attributed to reduced blood flow to the brain caused by age-related changes in the arteries that supply the head.
- Neurons are oxygen-sensitive and will not function when faced with a decline in the oxygen supply. They may die if the full oxygen supply is not restored.
- Loss of synapses may be more important than neuron losses.
- Synapses are vital for memory and learning.

The hippocampus and memory

- The hippocampal complex consists of the dentate gyrus and Ammon's horn, which is further divided into areas CA1, CA2, CA3 and CA4.
- The subiculum, the entorhinal cortex, the perirhinal cortex and the parahippocampal cortex are all areas of the temporal lobe linked to the hippocampus.

How memory works

- Memory is based on the formation of long-term potentiation (LTP) or long-term depression (LTD) at the synapse, leading to the formation of new synapses.
- Damage to Ammon's horn CA1 and CA3 areas, the fornix, the mammillary bodies and the anterior thalamic nucleus can cause memory loss.

Alzheimer disease

- Alzheimer disease is a dementia with the presence of extracellular plaques and intracellular neurofibrillary tangles.
- The early-age onset of AD is more genetically based than the late-age onset.
- The plaques have a central core of abnormal beta-amyloid protein (Aβ42).
- Familial Alzheimer disease (FAD) usually has mutations of the *APP* (chromosome 21), *PS-1* (chromosome 14), *PS-2* (chromosome 1) and *ERAB* (chromosome X) genes.
- The tangles inside the neurons are made from an abnormal form of tau protein.
- In the over-65 age group, 20–40% have a mutation of the ApoE (apolipoprotein E) gene on chromosome 19.
- AD may be inflammatory in nature and is possibly caused by the bacterium *Chlamydia pneumoniae* in some cases.
- AD is linked with Down syndrome through chromosome 21.

The drugs used in dementia

- Donepezil and rivastigmine are reversible acetylcholinesterase inhibitors that reduce the rate of cognitive deterioration in about 40% of cases.
- Ampakines are drugs for the future improvement of memory. They increase activity of the AMPA receptors that boost NMDA receptor function in memory and learning.

References

Bear M. F., Connors B. W. and Pardiso M. A. (1996) *Neuroscience: Exploring the Brain*. Williams and Wilkins, Baltimore.

Beardsley T. (1997) The machinery of thought. *Scientific American*, Aug: 58–63.

Bentley P. (1999) Dementia demystified. *Nursing Times*, **10** (95): 47–49.

Biernacki C. and Barratt J. (2001) Improving the nutritional status of people with dementia. *British Journal of Nursing*, **10** (17): 1104–1114.

Blows W. T. (2000) The nervous system, part 2. *Nursing Times*, **96** (40): 45–48.

Concar D. (1997) Brain boosters. *New Scientist*, 8 Feb.: 32–36.

Day S. (2002) Painful memories. *New Scientist*, **173** (2332; 2 March): 29–31.

Haines D. E. (1995) *Neuroanatomy, An Atlas of Structures, Sections and Systems* (4th edn). Williams and Wilkins, Baltimore.

Katzman R. and Kawas C. (1998) Risk factors for Alzheimer's disease. *Neuroscience News*, **1** (4): 27–34.

Maier-Lorentz M. M. (2000a) Neurobiological basis for Alzheimer's disease. *Journal of Neuroscience Nursing*, **32** (2): 117–125.

Maier-Lorentz M. M. (2000b) Effective nursing interventions for the management of Alzheimer's disease. *Journal of Neuroscience Nursing*, **32** (3): 153–157.

Roberts G. W., Leigh P. N. and Weinberger D. R. (1993) *Neuropsychiatric Disorders*. Wolfe, London.

Saftig P., Craessaerts K., Vanderstichele H., Guhde G., Annaert W., von Figura K., van Leuven F. and de Strooper B. (1998) The two major familial Alzheimer's disease gene products: presenilin 1 and amyloid precursor protein interact functionally. *Neuroscience News*, **1** (4): 35–38.

Schmidt M. L., Lee V. M., Forman M., Chiu T. S. and Trojanowski J. Q. (1997) Monoclonal antibodies to a 100-kd protein revealed abundant A beta-negative plaques throughout grey matter of Alzheimer's disease brains. *The American Journal of Pathology*, **151** (1): 69–80.

Smith D., Clark R., Jobst K. A., Sutton L., Ueland P. M. and Refsum H. (1998) Hyperhomocysteinemia: an independent risk factor for histopathologically-confirmed Alzheimer's disease, *in Homocysteine: A Possible Risk Factor for Alzheimer's Disease*, (http://www.sciencedaily.com/releases/1998/05/980504125421.htm).

OPTIMA (Oxford Project to Investigate Memory and Ageing), Oxford University.

Index

gangliosides 190
general anxiety disorder 146
generalised seizures 204, 207, 212, 217
generic drug name 113
gene expression 42, 64
genes 64, 74–7, 81
gene promoter 64
gene transcription 64, 141
genotype 100
german measles 88
ghosts 145
Gilles de la Tourette syndrome 92
glial cells (neuroglia) 22, 34–7
gliosis 34, 36, 250, 255
globus pallidus 11–13, 222, 223, 227
glossopharyngeal nerve 15
glucocorticoids 67
glutamate (glutamic acid) 32, 35, 48,
    49, 172, 223
glutamate pathways 48, 50
glutamate receptors 32, 48, 49
glutamic acid decarboxylase (GAD) 48,
    49
glutamine 233
glycine 52
glycolipids 190
GNAL gene 163
golgi apparatus (or body) 236
gonadotrophic hormones 87, 176
grand mal seizures 204, 209, 212, 213,
    217
granulocytes 191
grey matter 3, 34
growth hormone 10, 176
guanine 77
gustatory area 243
gustatory hallucinations 215
gyrus (gyri) 3, 87, 241, 242

half life (of a drug) 111, 116
hallucinations 130, 159, 160, 167, 225
hallucinogenic drugs 130
haloperidol 92, 174, 176
Harvey's disease 235–7
heart block 195
hemispheres (of cerebrum) 7
heroin (diamorphine) 117
herpes virus 199
heterozygous alleles 75
high density lipoprotein (HDL) 190,
    191
hippocampus 8, 125, 138, 142, 161,
    165–7, 242–4, 246
Hirano bodies 255
histadine 60
histadine decarboxylase 60
histamine 60

histamine pathways 61
histamine receptors 60
homeostasis 65
homocysteine 253
homologous chromosomes 75
homovanillic acid 43, 171
homozygous alleles 75
hormone receptors 63
hormones 33, 63–73, 187
5-HT 1A receptor gene 163
5-HT 2A receptor gene 162
human immunodeficiency virus (HIV)
    120, 128, 177
humoral immunity 189, 190
huntingtin protein 232–4
huntingtin-associated protein 1 (HAP-1)
    232–4
Huntington disease (HD) 79, 81, 231–5
H-Y antigen 96, 97
hydrocephalus 87, 88
hydrogen peroxide 251, 252
4-hydroxy-3-methoxymethamphetamine
    (HMMA) 123
5-hydroxyindoleacetic acid (5-HIAA)
    47
11β-hydroxylase 68
21-hydroxylase 68
5-hydroxytryptamine (5-HT, serotonin)
    46, 118, 148–50, 184, 185
5-hydroxytryptophan 47
hyperammonaemia 91
hypercalciuria 236
hypergraphia 215
hypermetamorphosis 147
hyperphagia 87
hyperphosphorylation 252
hyperplasia 68
hypertension 141, 147, 197
hyperthermia 127
hyperthyroid (thyrotoxicosis) 66
hypofrontality 167
hypoglossal nerve 15
hypogonadism 87, 102
hypokinesia 224
hyponatraemia 195
hypoplasia 102
hypotension 113, 176, 230
hypothalamo-pituitary-adrenal (HPA)
    axis 66, 147, 187, 188, 198
hypothalamo-pituitary-thyroid (HPT)
    axis 66, 188
hypothalamus 3, 10, 53, 54, 70, 137,
    140, 147, 176
hypothermia 176
hypothyroid disorders (myxoedema) 65,
    66, 187
hypotonia 86